SEPARATED ANGELS

SHANNON *and* MEGAN

the FANNING *twins*

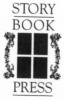

STORY
BOOK

PRESS

Book Design & Consulting:
Absolute Impressions
Downers Grove, IL

Cover Design:
BrainTrust
Chicago, IL

Editing:
Leanne Pankuch
Sandi Fanning

Illustrations:
Laura Fanning

Photo:
Jennifer Wolfe Photography
Downers Grove, IL

Storybook Press, Inc.
PO Box 4438,
Naperville, Illinois 60540

Printed in the United States of America

ISBN 0-9646812-0-X

Dedication

To all my family and friends, whose encouragement
and help has made the production of this book possible,
to my partner Sandi, and all of our beautiful children,
and to my lovely sisters Jeanette Fanning Anderson and
Dorothy Fanning O'Donnell.

Forward

*It is common for people to seek extension of their own
existence through their offspring. When the well being,
and even the very lives of those same offspring are in
danger, however, it is only too easy to understand the
true frailty of such existence. Man was given both heart and
soul to help understand these situations, and to respond
in whatever way is best; not for himself,
but for the children, born or unborn.*

CHAPTER 1

Mixed Emotions

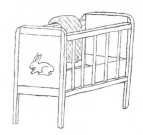

I can't say that the possibility of fathering twins never crossed my mind. The fact is, I had actually thought about it any number of times.

You see, my youngest brother and sister are twins, my older sister has identical twin boys, and up until recently I, like many other people, believed that twins of either variety were hereditary. Still, I could have, in no way, expected that this particular set of twins would so dramatically impact my life.

Sandi's situation was similar. Her family also has a history of twins. But, at the time we were first married, she possessed a greater knowledge of how and why they happened than I did. In the end it mattered very little; we were both just part of the marvelous miracle.

Our story is one of love, trust, and faith. To relate it properly, I must provide a little history.

Sandi and I were both previously married, she for seven years and I for twenty-seven. As you might have guessed, there is a notable difference in our ages. Chronologically, it is more than thirteen years.

I am from a rather large family, having been born tenth out of thirteen children. Sandi, on the other hand, is one of two children.

I have three grown children of my own, two girls and a boy. All are over the age of 22. Sandi has two young daughters, aged 4 and 9.

From the very beginning, the age factor did not seem to be a problem. Sandi and I think very much alike, and enjoy most of the same activities. We even share a great number of likes and dislikes, including those regarding food, music and sports.

When we had known each other for just over a year and a half, we decided to marry. Preparations began almost immediately. There was little difficulty involved in determining where and when; the how turned out to be a bit of a problem, though. We wanted the service to be simple, but special. Eventually we settled all the necessary details and prepared for the big event.

Sandi and I were married at a charming little church in Lombard, Illinois. Our wedding was very special, for a number of reasons. First of all, the previously mentioned age difference. Also, Sandi's soon-to-be eight year old daughter was the maid of honor. The wedding took place on a Sunday, (the first time in either of our families). And possibly most memorable of all, was the fact that a number of different people sang at the service. This included friends, coworkers and family members (my brother, my daughter and myself). It was one of the best planned, happiest and yet most nerve-racking experiences I had ever known.

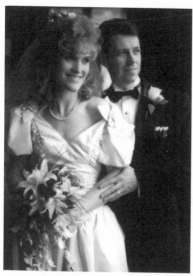

Sandi and I on our wedding day.
We had no idea what lie ahead.
Photo by Jennifer Wolfe

Following the wedding, things began to settle in rather nicely. My children readily accepted Sandi, and her daughters seemed to have few problems adjusting to their new environment. In fact, we were all getting used to and enjoying our enlarged family.

Prior to the wedding, Sandi had informed me of her desire to have another child. She had said she would really like to have a boy she could dress-up in all those cute little boy clothes. Since my son Paul was 22 years old, he would not fit the bill.

I was a little concerned. With my children being grown, I was prepared to focus more on the joys of grandparenting. Since I already had 3 grandchildren, it seemed only appropriate. Deciding it was necessary for me to do some strong self examination before making a commitment, I spent a lot of time going over all of the pluses and minuses, and there were a number of each. My three children were now grown. I was able to do just about as I pleased with my spare time, and there was a lot more of it than there had been when they were small. On the other hand, I did miss having little ones around the house, and sharing in the joy of watching them develop. This decision, it seemed, would not be an easy one.

The more I thought about it, however, the better the idea sounded. It would be very interesting to see what sort of offspring the two of us could produce.

I remember jokingly acknowledging that, although we had to keep the other five children we already had (trade and/or sale being illegal) it wouldn't hurt, and might actually be fun to have another little face at the kitchen table.

It was, therefore, with full agreement that we began our efforts at enlarging the family. Sandi had set up a plan so that our attempts would take place on the appropriate days, when her body temperature was just where it needed to be. Apparently, that's one of the indicators that "the time is right."

I don't know how well this method works overall, but for us, it appeared to be an almost immediate success. Within a few weeks of the day we started, Sandi tested positive in a home examination. We were very pleased and anxious to make sure everything went just right. She immediately set up an appointment with her friend and Obstetrician/Gynecologist, Meghan Flannery.

Sandi had met Meghan when they were both students at Millikin University. Although Meghan had gone on to become a doctor and Sandi to become an engineer, they had managed to stay in touch. Meghan now had and office just a few minutes from where we lived in Naperville, Illinois.

When first visiting Meghan's office, we were both in very good humor and anxious for some information about

Sandi's condition. The news received, however, turned out to be far from good. There appeared to be some irregularities in the pregnancy.

Meghan wanted to run some additional tests right away. There is a certain hormone, identified as HCG, whose concentration should double in a 48 hour period of normal pregnancy. Sandi was tested for the hormone's presence, with unencouraging results. The level had increased in the 48 hours, but had not doubled. It seemed from then on that one bit of bad news led to another. This was not turning out to be the happy event we had been hoping for.

Meghan thought that, because of the slow growth in hormone levels, the pregnancy might be ectopic. I had heard this term before, but had no idea of what it applied to. It was explained to me that ectopic meant the egg may have implanted in the fallopian tube, rather than the uterus.

An ultrasound was performed, and we were given more reason for concern. At such an early point in the pregnancy, the test should have shown a small black dot, representing the embryonic sac. A black dot did appear, but it was even smaller than it should have been.

Meghan explained to us that the next step should be a laparoscopy on Sandi to determine for certain whether or not it was a tubal pregnancy. We agreed, and it was performed almost immediately. The procedure turned out to be somewhat painful, and the results were negative.

Doctor Flannery decided to continue to monitor Sandi rather closely. She was now almost certain that the pregnancy was not normal. We kept hoping and praying that she was wrong, that everything would turn out okay.

Meghan, however, had been correct. Within two weeks nature took over and Sandi miscarried.

She was understandably upset. It was several weeks before either one of us even felt like talking about trying again. When we did, she was as positive as ever. She approached me rather gently regarding the subject, however; sensing, I guess, that I might have changed my mind.

I, on the other hand, knowing how badly she had wanted the baby, yet fearful of the possibilities for more heartbreak, began to re-evaluate the decision to have another child. Were we being sent a message? Should we abandon our attempts at increasing the family?

I performed more soul searching, and came to believe that there was a message for us, and I knew just what it was. Someone upstairs wanted us to have another child, but first, they wanted to make sure we realized how special it would be, and how much hurt could take place when it didn't happen as we had planned. I realized that many couples go through this more than once. They must be very strong indeed. This one, single loss hurt an awful lot. I knew then, more than ever before, how lucky and wonderful it is to have even one healthy child.

I told Sandi that when the time was right, we should try again. She happily agreed, and we renewed our efforts. The wait, once more, was not long. Within a few short weeks, the home testing kit again indicated Sandi was pregnant.

Prior to Sandi getting pregnant, we had planned a trip to Colorado to see my mother and sisters. They had seen

Sandi only once, that being prior to the wedding. We felt the trip would be good for all of us. The plan was to leave in early September, and to drive all the way. Meghan didn't see any reason for us to change our plans.

Once she had known we were trying again, she prearranged for the hormone test to be performed as soon as we thought pregnancy was likely. This was to be followed up by early ultrasound examination. The bloodwork for the HCG could take place immediately, but the results would not be back for several days.

We were, therefore, in Colorado when we received the call from Meghan's office. The results looked much better. In fact, the hormone level had not just doubled, it had quadrupled. Upon hearing this, Sandi and I looked at each other and, at the same time, and said "Twins!". Of course, as far as we knew, there was no correlation between the quadrupling of the hormone and a twin pregnancy. At the time, we thought we were just adding a little humor to the, so far happy, situation. My mother, on the other hand, thought that twins would be only appropriate. She had given birth to my youngest brother and sister when she was in her forties. There was now reason why I shouldn't follow her lead, by fathering my own set. We had to explain to her that we had been joking, and, as far as anyone knew right now, we were only having one.

When we returned home, we began to concentrate more seriously on the pregnancy. It seemed as though things were happening rather quickly. The initial ultrasound was set to take place about 8 weeks into the pregnancy. We could hardly wait. After the last series of ultrasonic tests, I was just a bit apprehensive; not enough, however, to overcome my anticipation and excitement.

There hadn't been an ultrasound examination performed on my first wife for any of our children. I don't believe the technology even existed back then. The first pregnancy ultrasound I had ever seen was that performed on Sandi during our first pregnancy together. I had found it rather amazing, even though, at that stage of gestation, there was little to see. I could hardly wait for this one. I knew it would show a lot more.

I went with Sandi, of course, and we were both somewhat nervous at the start. Linda, one of the partners in Meghan's practice, was the technician. She had been very good with us during our previous experiences there. She was very friendly and quite competent. The procedure she had previously followed, was to start the examination, see how everything looked, and then call in Doctor Flannery to have a look. It appeared as though it was going to be about the same this time.

Sandi lay back on the table with her head cocked so as to see the examination screen for herself. As Linda began gently probing to locate some telltale sign (a tiny heartbeat or a more noticeable head) I questioned her as to what "we" should be looking for. She didn't seem to mind the question, and began explaining.

Just as she described what a heart would look like, a tiny blinking beacon appeared on the center left portion of the screen. At about the same instant, a second beacon appeared only a fraction of a centimeter from the first. Sandi and I hardly had time to look at one and other.

Again, as with one voice, we said "twins!!"

Linda seemed a little surprised, but remained rather calm considering the situation. Of course she had probably been through this sort of thing any number of times. She admitted that there did indeed seem to be two hearts; then, after looking a little closer, decided to go get Doctor Flannery.

It wasn't long before Linda returned to the room with Meghan. Doctor Flannery's reaction was similar to what Linda's had been. She was calm and guarded. We could understand that. She must have wanted to make absolutely sure of what we were seeing. She could probably already tell by our faces, that Sandi and I were overjoyed. This examination had been everything I expected and more. Seeing those two tiny lives, just beginning, yet already recognizable, convinced me that creation really is marvelous and miraculous.

Some time was spent probing with the ultrasound to try and get a more accurate picture of the pregnancy. As far as we could tell, the only things it really showed us were two small hearts and two small heads. There were two!

We spent the remainder of our visit time talking with Meghan about the meaning of what we had seen. She was very nice and told us what she could. She then explained that she believed, because of the circumstances, it would be better for us to see another doctor; one that specialized in high risk pregnancies. She recommended a group out of Lutheran General in Park Ridge. Before we left her office, she provided us with their names and telephone number as well. There was not a lot more she could do for us at that time, but she did want us to think it over for a day or two, and call with any questions and/or problems we might have.

When we heard the term "high risk," it scared us a little. We still were not sure why, all of a sudden, this pregnancy would be considered more risky than any other. Meghan had explained to us that many doctors consider any multiple embryo pregnancy to be high risk, but that, in itself, did not seem like enough reason. The next day, back at Meghan's office, we received some additional clarification.

It wasn't just the multiple embryos. The doctor could tell by the close proximity of the hearts to one another, and the identification of only one sack, that these two babies were extremely close to each other; most likely occupying the same sack. They explained to us that there were several serious problems with a shared sack. First of all, the babies would be in double danger. If anything happened to one, the other would be effected almost immediately. Secondly, it would be very easy for one baby to get entangled in the cord of the other, or even worse, for both babies to become entangled. Any sort of entanglement could mean disaster. Lastly, there was even a possibility our babies were attached to one another, or conjoined.

Now we really became concerned. We began asking questions about the statistics concerning the problems with single sack twins. We did not press the issue of them being conjoined right away, as we knew that the likelihood of this occurrence was very low due to the known rarity.

The statistics on survival of twins in the same sack

pointed to a rate of only about 50 percent. This news was almost heartbreaking, and certainly very difficult for us to accept. Sandi and I became of a single mindset. These babies would survive, statistically probable or not.

After a few minutes of thought and discussion, we came back to the statement regarding the possibility of the twins being conjoined. We knew what this meant. Many people still referred to such twins as "Siamese." We preferred the term conjoined. Was it really possible though? Wasn't this the sort of thing that only happened to other families? We needed to have more information. How many times had they seen ultrasounds like this turn out to represent conjoined twins? What percentage of babies sharing a sack turned out to be this way? What percentage of pregnancies ended up in conjoined twins? What was the survival rate in those cases?

The answers to our questions came quickly. They did not have any statistics on conjoined twins. They had never performed an ultrasound with similar results, and had never been involved with a pregnancy that was diagnosed this way. Perhaps the doctors in Lutheran General's high risk group would be able to tell us more. Meghan and Sandi set up an appointment for the next available time slot.

Approximately one week later, we were on our way to Park Ridge, and Lutheran General Hospital, to see the high risk-pregnancy specialists. We were both nervous and apprehensive.

The drive there took long enough that Sandi and I managed to say a rosary, before carrying on a rather lengthy conversation. Of the five children we had between us, none had been considered in any way to have been in danger prior to birth; at least, no more than in any normal pregnancy. We had no real idea what to expect, although the long drive gave us time to develop some pretty good notions.

First impressions, thank goodness, are not always accurate and telling. We know that the doctors at Lutheran General are professional and caring; and that they hold life in the highest esteem. The first day we met them, however we didn't know all these things. That visit was a painful one, and will be remembered for a very long time.

We had made it clear from the beginning that I wanted to be present for any testing that took place, unless this was just not possible. The staff at Lutheran General didn't seem to mind much, so I waited patiently with Sandi, while they prepared her for another ultrasound. Being in the engineering field by profession, and knowing something about ultrasonics, it was easy for us to notice, while waiting, that the hospital had some pretty sophisticated equipment.

I got the idea that most practices must work about the same when it comes to ultrasonic examinations. Lutheran General didn't seem to be much different than Meghan's office. The technician set up the patient, adjusted the equipment, and performed some measuring and preliminary probing. When the doctor arrived, the technician continued under his direction. Eventually, the doctor took the transducer himself and continued probing and evaluating.

The specific Doctor we had been referred to was Bruce Pielet. When we arrived, however, he was tied up with another patient; so one of the other doctors began the examination. He spent quite a bit of time probing ultra-sonically before instructing us to wait for Doctor Pielet, who would be there in a few minutes. Following him, two additional technicians were called in to view the screen and provide input.

I was certainly no expert on this type of ultrasound examination. Nonetheless, I had my face as close to the monitor as possible in an attempt to see whatever was there, and help us make our own evaluation. In the position Sandi was forced to maintain, it was almost impossible for her to watch the screen.

The examination went on for much longer than I had expected. When it was completed, we still seemed to have the same unanswered questions. The doctors and technicians left us then, to converse privately about what they had just seen.

From the conversation that had taken place while we were in the ultrasound room, we knew that Doctor Pielet believed that the twins were indeed joined in the area of the abdomen; just how severely he could not tell. If the pregnancy continued, he would be able to learn much more in the weeks ahead.

The other doctor went along with Doctor Pielet, who seemed to be the expert. There was, however, something else he saw which caused him to offer an even more heartbreaking prognosis. When the doctors and technicians had finished their conversation, he came into the private room where we had been waiting.

He was polite but frank in speech and mannerism, and his comments really hit home.

It wasn't enough to hear that the experts believed that

our babies were joined. Now, this doctor told us that he had noticed a "shadowed" area around the neck and head of one baby. His guess was that this represented fluid. This was an indication that the baby was already experiencing difficulty, and was, he believed, in fetal stress.

We needed to know just what this "fetal stress" meant. How serious a situation did this represent? Neither of us had actually heard the term before, but it sounded quite ominous. I asked point blank, "just what does this mean? What should we expect."

He answered quite directly "It is my opinion that when you return in two weeks, one baby will be dead and the other will be dying."

We had realized we might receive some bad news, but this was about the worst. It was now impossible to keep the tears back. Sandi squeezed my hand tightly and said "I can see them move; I can't believe they're dying." All I could do was ask the doctor if he was positive. He reiterated the fact that he had given his professional opinion, and we were welcome to get additional opinions. We said we would like a little time to think about it.

In the meantime, it was necessary for him to present us with the options available. There were basically three:

1. Terminate the pregnancy immediately.
2. Allow nature to take it's course (miscarriage would take place within 6 weeks if the doctor was correct).
3. Continue with the pregnancy, monitor closely and make decisions based on ultrasounds and other tests.

We chose 3, realizing that if the doctor was right, it wouldn't really matter. The last thing he said to us that day was, "I don't want you leaving this office believing that you have a normal conjoined pregnancy." Nothing anyone could have said would've made us feel any worse.

We made a follow-up appointment for a couple of weeks later, and left the doctor's office. The walk back to our van was quiet and rather long, neither of us really knowing what to say. Once in the privacy of our own vehicle, however, we cried and comforted one and other.

Chapter 2

An Adjusted Prognosis

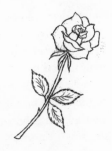

The two weeks that followed were difficult for us to say the least. It seemed as though I was asking Sandi how she felt every hour or so. Was there any discomfort? Had anything changed? She was being very positive, and telling me she felt just fine. Both of us were working full time each day, and sleeping poorly each night. We continued, of course, to discuss the situation with one and other. Each time, our opinions were as one. We would continue with the pregnancy as long as possible, and gather as much information about conjoined twins as we could. Our decisions would be based on what the ultrasounds and other tests showed, with additional information being used as reference data. We both really wanted these babies. We prayed to God each day that the doctor was wrong, and our babies would live.

Sandi is a real good-news type person. She doesn't like to talk a lot if what she has to relate is negative. The situation is much different, however, when there is positive news to be shared. She wants to tell everyone she knows.

Because of the earlier miscarriage, I had been rather

hesitant in spreading the good news about this latest pregnancy. I guess I was worried about how we would handle if something else wasn't quite right. Sandi, however, had not been so worried, and had wanted to tell a number of people just as soon as we were sure she was pregnant. We had eventually agreed that we would wait until the results of the hormone test had been received and had shown a normal increase.

There were a good number of friends and relatives who were quite happy to hear that our family was going to expand. Some of these folks worked with or for us. This meant that once the results of the hormone test were known, virtually all of our associates knew we were having a baby. Once the pregnancy was diagnosed as "high risk", going to work each day became a much more difficult proposition. Most of these other individuals were genuinely concerned about what was happening with our family. Updating them on the situation and repeating the painful parts so often during that 2 week period, provided us with our own personal torture.

I realized, looking at it from a positive viewpoint, there may also have been some additional benefits to the situation at work. As I previously mentioned, we both worked in an engineering department during this time. I found that it really helped when I utilized some of the same type of logic in my thoughts about the pregnancy, as in my work duties. Not only did this tend to remove some of the emotional stress, but looking at the situation from a more technical standpoint helped me to analyze and better understand what was happening.

For instance, I realized a similarity between a doctor's evaluation of a medical situation and an engineer's evaluation of a design. In both cases the individual utilizes past experience, education and reference literature; but in the long run, each has to rely on his or her own judgment to determine what it all means. Having known some very fine engineers to be wrong upon occasion, we saw no reason to preclude the idea that the doctor might just have made a judgment error. This, of course fit in very well with the positive position we had both taken. Besides, engineers like to have as many facts as possible before developing theories or conclusions. We might have to respect the doctor's opinion, and even try to understand why he believed as he did, but we certainly did not have to agree with him. Not yet!

The days continued to pass slowly. We looked for everything positive we could find to help get us through this first emotional trial. We became involved in much longer discussions about our babies than had been planned or expected. It seemed as though we were possibly unknowingly seeking to get as much support as possible for our decision. We really wanted others to tell us we were doing the right thing, even though we felt it was our best and only choice.

The support, thankfully, was there. Our friends and relatives, if they commented at all, said they would have made the same choice. Although these comments may not have done a lot to ease the emotional strain, they were, at least, heartwarming. Particularly when coming from close family members.

Following our last visit to Doctor Flannery's office, Sandi and I had discussed the pregnancy with my oldest daughter Leanne. When she heard about the ultrasound, she expressed a strong interest in seeing it herself. Just coincidentally, Meghan had offered to copy it for us on videotape, and we had agreed. I had thought, at the time, it would be nice for some of Sandi's close friends to see. For me, of course, it had acted as documented proof of the miracle of conception.

Leanne's husband, Ray, was also interested in seeing the tape. So, the next time they came to visit, we took the time to run it through the VCR.

The ultrasound itself had affected me rather profoundly, from an emotional standpoint. That was to be expected. After all, I was the father. It didn't seem reasonable, however, to assume that others would be similarly affected.

I was a bit surprised, therefore, when I saw Leanne's reaction. Both her and Ray had definitely been affected. One look at their eyes told the whole story. They were full of love and wonder.

I don't remember what was said from that point on, but whatever it was, it sure made us feel good. They were very positive and supportive of our viewpoint. Leanne said that when she saw the babies on the tape, they were so very alive and real, that she immediately knew how we felt, and that we had been right in our decision. Ray also voiced his support, and commented on how moved he had been by the video.

That one evening presented us with enough additional support to help lift any shadow of a doubt which may have begun to descend on us. We were doing the right thing, and, with God's help, we would see the proof the following spring.

By the time of our second visit to Lutheran General ,we were physically and mentally tired, as well as being rather drained emotionally. Although we had remained positive, it was impossible to prevent ourselves from thinking about the possibilities of a negative outcome. Nothing had changed as far as we could tell. Sandi felt the same as she had when we visited two weeks earlier. If one of the babies had died, then it must not have been possible to tell this early in the pregnancy. I supposed we would have to wait until Sandi's body began ridding itself of the dead tissue. We chose to believe simply that nothing had happened. On the way to Lutheran General, we said a rosary together, hoping that someone higher up might see fit to influence the day's outcome in a positive manner.

We entered the doctors' office with a slightly different attitude that day. The first time there we had been anxious to get their opinion; this time were anxious to disprove that same opinion.

We nervously waited for Sandi's turn. The wait was not long. Once again she was to receive an extensive ultrasonic examination. This time, however, she would first be examined as if this were a normal pregnancy.

All of the preliminaries were performed by a nurse. She treated Sandi very well, and acted as she might with any other patient. This did strike me as a little odd. Based on what had been said during our last appointment, it would have seemed as though they might consider these activities a waste of time.

The nurse then moved Sandi to an ultrasound room, where she was prepared for examination. At that point, I could actually feel my wife's apprehension, and was sure she could feel mine as well. We knew enough about this type of examination to know it would tell us if one of our babies had indeed died.

It seemed as though all of the emotions of the past weeks were coming to a head. All the fears, hopes and prayers we had shared were so very clear in my mind. I wanted to get the whole examination over with. More than that, however, I wanted to see two healthy heartbeats.

As the technician attached the transducer and positioned it over Sandi's stomach, I moved as close as I could to my wife. Whatever we would see, we would see it together.

By now we were fairly familiar with the procedure. The transducer was "slid" over the jelly which had been applied to the surface of the skin. At the same time, the technician watched the monitor, to determine just how the babies were positioned. It seemed to be taking longer to find the babies than before. I hoped the technician was just being more careful.

Suddenly, we saw two distinctive shapes, easily identifiable as heads. Before I could determine just what this meant, she moved the transducer down the stomach and over toward the side. Almost instantaneously the profile of two tiny bodies appeared, and just as quickly, two heartbeats. I was thrilled. I tightened the grip on Sandi's hand even as I felt the pressure of her own grip increase. She had seen them also. I knew that we had only just begun a long and difficult journey, that there might still be much pain ahead for us, but I was happy and thankful for this gift. I took the time to whisper "thank you Lord."

The ultrasound was, once again, a very long one. When the technician had finished all of the preliminaries (measurements and body part identification) Doctor Pielet took over. He spent a considerable amount of time examining the area at which he believed the fetuses to be joined. His opinion did not change. He was now, in fact, even more sure. Thankfully though, they were still both very much alive. The doctor had been, at least partially, wrong.

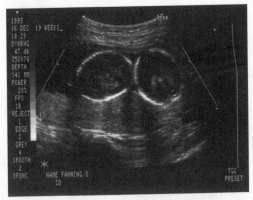

Early ultrasounds revealed two heads very close together, but definitely separate.
Luthern General Perinatal Center

As I said before, I was not an ultrasound expert. There were some things, however, which could be easily picked out by an amateur like me. One of these was the shaded area, believed by the doctor, to represent fluid. This "shadow" appeared around the neck/head area of one of the babies just as it had during our last visit. I had noticed it then even before the doctor had pointed it out; and it appeared to be no different now than it was then at the time I had first seen it. I wondered if it might not have been the outline of the sack which contains the baby and surrounding fluid. Now I was wondering just what other possibilities there might be.

Since the examination was being performed by Doctor Pielet this time, I would question him on this issue when the time was appropriate. Upon completion of the examination, we were again taken into a private room to wait for the doctor. The wait was probably very short. With the situation as it was, however, it seemed almost like forever.

This time Doctor Pielet saw us alone. I remember that Sandi and I had shared the same opinion of him following our first visit. He had appeared quite professional and somewhat cold, with no sense of humor. (We had attempted to use mild and tasteful humor to both break the ice and relieve some of the tension). With Doctor Pielet it had not worked. He began the conversation much as we had expected. He was even more sure the babies were joined now. It was not, however, an absolute. If we continued with the pregnancy, we should know more as the weeks passed. Had we made any decision yet?

Sandi answered right away. We were continuing with the pregnancy. At her reply, the doctor was neither upset nor in any way excited. It seemed as though he had only asked the question to help determine what the next step should be.

He went on to explain how it was not really critical at this point. Termination could actually still take place up to twenty-four weeks. He explained, in more detail, what kind of testing could be performed at what particular stages of the pregnancy to help us get all of the facts. He then began to talk more about what to expect should the babies indeed be joined.

I couldn't wait any longer. I had to ask him about the other doctor's original prognosis? I explained to Doctor Pielet about the "shadow" area of fluid around one of the baby's neck. "I'm not seeing that," he stated.

This was more than a bit surprising. The one item which we had been told was evidential of the twins demise, was now not even noticeable! Or was the truth that he had never really thought that it was fluid in the first place?

I began to explain how Sandi and I had been worrying, waiting, hoping, praying, etc. for almost 2 weeks. All I got out was "we have..." Doctor Pielet, apparently thinking I was about to say something else, finished my sentence for me. "We have a difference of opinion on that issue."

What did this mean? Was he indeed saying that he had never thought the babies were in fetal stress? Apparently so!

As the conversation continued, he confirmed it for us. He had not interpreted the "shadow" to indicate fetal stress.

Sandi and I looked at each other. Again our emotions took over. We were relieved, yet apprehensive. Hopeful but angry. It seemed we had been through an awful lot unnecessarily. We almost didn't know how to react. Our immediate prayers for the babies had been answered.

Doctor Pielet continued where he had left off regarding possibilities and options. Should the babies be joined, there were a good number of scenarios to be considered. They may share one or more vital organs. One baby may have all organs and be fully functional, while the other is lacking any number of different organs. And, there was always the possibility that they shared only skin and some muscle tissue. The last, based on the ultrasounds, seemed to be the least likely.

By this time, it seemed that the possibility of the twins not being joined at all had faded into impossibility. We brought it up, and were reminded that having two babies this close in a single sack carried a low survival probability. We would continue being positive, and hoping for the very best of all possible outcomes. In the meantime, we had to start thinking about which way we might go when the decision times came. In our minds, of course, there would continue to be only one right way to go, but we knew even the best road might contain a fork or two.

Sandi and I believed we needed to know as much about all the possibilities as anyone could tell us, and Doctor Pielet agreed. He related to us basically what to expect and what to look for. He talked to us about the number of important decisions along the way.

The steps to be taken were simple to start with: Continue close monitoring of the pregnancy, with regular ultrasounds and probably an eventual MRI.

As for the issue of what organs, vital or otherwise, might be shared, the discussion was brief. We could get more information on that subject as necessary. For now, we knew the basics. Obviously, the sharing of single organs after separation was not possible. Kidneys could, for instance be divided; heart, stomach and others could not. A single liver might, depending on circumstances, be successfully "split" in two.

Now that we were in agreement with the doctor about continuation of the pregnancy, all seemed a bit more relaxed. Doctor Pielet seemed to warm to us a little, and began explaining what was required of Sandi as an expectant mother of twins. Things still were far from normal, but at least the focus had shifted a little.

We concluded our second visit having a more substantial plan than we came with. It was by no means positive that the twins were out of the woods as far as fetal stress or other complications were concerned, but we now had a better idea of what we should be looking for, and when decisions might be required.

Before we left the office, Sandi made it clear to Doctor Pielet that she did not wish to be examined by the other doctor again. I was upset with him as well, but couldn't keep from remembering the engineering comparison. He had used his experience and knowledge to formulate an opinion. It looked as though he had guessed wrong.

On the way home that day, Sandi related some of her thoughts to me. "Maybe," she said, "the babies are just slightly joined at the abdomen so that they cannot move enough to get tangled with one another. It might turn out to be a blessing in disguise." This sounded good to me and I told her so. It gave us something a little more positive to focus on.

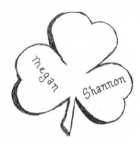

CHAPTER 3

Preparing for What?

It doesn't really matter how many children you already have. When you receive the news that your family is about to increase, the urge, if not the need, to acquire new baby "things" becomes quite strong. This pregnancy was no different. We knew that the clothes and other necessities Sandi had left over from her youngest would not be enough for two new babies; and virtually everything that had been purchased for any of my other children was long since gone. When we tried planning what to get, however, we found the desire to follow through and go out and shop just wasn't there. It seemed as though we were concerned that if we got everything for the twins ahead of time, we might be "jinxing" them. It sounds pretty foolish; but remember, both times we had rushed out to announce the pregnancy, things had taken a turn for the worse. Following our first visit to Lutheran General, we had quietly ceased all such activity. This included one of my favorite baby related functions, choosing names.

I have my own (rather strong) opinions on this subject. I believe most people do not put enough thought into naming, especially from their children's viewpoint. That's why so many youngsters grow up unhappy with their names. Some mothers-to-be show a real lack of logic when it comes to name choosing; and the fathers may be even worse.

Some fathers can't be bothered by the effort required, and just let the mother choose a name, provided it is sensible. Some apparently don't care if it is sensible or not. And others wait to see what she chooses so that they can argue about it. I would like to believe that the majority of fathers-to-be, however, are more like me; and actually enjoy going through books and lists of names hour after hour in hopes of finding just the right match.

Since Sandi and I had known early on that we could expect two, we began looking for matching pairs of names before her ninth week. The initial news we received from Lutheran General slowed this activity down considerably, even stopping it altogether for a period of time. We had found two boys' names that we agreed on rather quickly, but the continued search for girls names only tended to add more hills to the emotional roller coaster ride we had been experiencing. Even though our attitudes and outlooks were positive, a rest from such activities was necessary.

Sandi and I received much support from family and friends throughout those difficult times. There were so many helpful people that we probably never even thanked most of them. My own family certainly fell into this category. They were nothing but helpful and positive from the beginning. My sister Helen was constantly calling and/or stopping by to see how things were going. When she had first heard Sandi was pregnant, she promised to hold a baby shower. I had told her it wasn't' necessary, as we had both been married before and had children of various ages. She said "nonsense, this is your first child together, and she's family now. Remember, you are going to need a lot of new things." Sandi's mother had offered help in making some items for the baby's room, as did a couple of her friends. It seemed everyone wanted us to be prepared, and was willing to help. The problem was we really didn't know what to prepare for. This made it rather difficult to accept anyone's offer of assistance.

There was, of course much more preparation than that involving babies' names and clothes and the like. We had to be prepared for any and all of the possible outcomes. It would be necessary to make hard decisions along the way. The only way to be fully prepared was to know as much about conjoined twins and all of the associated problems, concerns and statistics as we possibly could.

The only information available at the local library was on twins or multiple births. Sandi already had many such books. These only barely, if ever, mentioned conjoined twins. They had helped verify some of what we had been told regarding single sack twins.

We realized we would have to find information elsewhere. Perhaps Lutheran General would be of some help to us.

Our next visit to see Doctor Pielet and crew was a bit more relaxed and a lot more like a pregnant woman should expect. It was plain to see that since the decision had been made to continue the pregnancy, they were going to make sure it was handled the best possible way. The staff was very pleasant yet professional. Sandi had to do all the normal things required of a pregnant woman. The ultrasound examination was the only out-of-the-ordinary activity. As we had expected, it was again very long and involved several different doctors and technicians.

Following the examination, we again spoke with Doctor Pielet. He seemed even a little warmer than before, and took some more time answering additional questions we had come up with. He offered to help find more information for us to read, and put us in touch with someone at the hospital who might also help. The only real change in the prognosis that day, was that he now believed the twins shared at least a liver, and possibly more. The probability that they were joined had grown.

We were not getting all of the positive results we had been hoping for. But, by the same token, they were not as negative as could have been the case either.

The examinations over the next few weeks did little more than add to the probability that our babies were joined. The ultrasounds showed nothing new, and the babies positions in regards to one and other never really changed. Over the same period of time, however, our knowledge on the subject of twins grew considerably. I had already known as much as, and maybe even more than most men about the conception process. By the time our pregnancy reached the fourth month, however, I knew far more than most anyone (not in the medical field) about all problems, conditions and possibilities regarding twins. This included the likelihood of conjoined twins and the survival rate of the same.

There had been a recent case in the news within our own geographical area involving twin girls. The media had covered this case rather closely, and we had watched with more than just passing interest. In addition, there just happened to have been two television specials concerning two other sets of conjoined twins. We watched these, and wrote down information and questions we thought might be of use to us later on. This included the names of doctors and hospitals we might need to contact.

One of the most interesting pieces of information was a list of fifty sets of conjoined twins. The list identified the date of birth, the manner in which they were joined, the action that was taken in each case, and the long range outcome. After reading the entire literature several times, we were not very uplifted. The number of incidents where both twins survived was low. The number with both twins fully functional at the age of twelve was heartbreaking.

We began to get a greater sense of just how unusual this pregnancy might be. Incidents of conjoined twins being conceived could be anywhere from one in one hundred thousand to one in two hundred thousand. Incidents of these twins surviving to reach birth might be as low as one in three hundred and fifty thousand. The reason for these figures being so imprecise were simple. Many pregnancies of this nature end in miscarriage. The fact that there were conjoined twins involved may have never been known. Also, because of problems which arise, some pregnancies are intentionally terminated early on.

Surviving the pregnancy is one thing; surviving the separation and subsequent recovery period quite another. Our best hope in this regard was to have the twins joined in a fashion dissimilar from any of those we had read about or seen on TV. The simple truth was that not a one case we knew of had been successful enough that both children ended up with a full set of functioning organs. Worse yet, was the fact that in less than 50% of the cases, had both twins even survived for more than a few short years.

Having both children healthy and complete had been important to us, but we now realized that having both of them alive was the more urgent need. Our thoughts began to turn toward the surgery that would almost certainly have to take place sometime after the twins were born.

We had attempted to use information gathering to help subdue any emotional upheavals we might experience. We wanted to be strong and positive all of the time. The best way to accomplish this, was to keep our minds fully occupied. Some of the time it worked, and some of the time it didn't. Every time we prayed or went to a church service, each time someone asked how it was going, and whenever we got in the van and headed for Park Ridge, our thoughts completely turned to our babies.

Doctor Pielet had, by the time Sandi was in her 15th week, performed five ultrasound examinations. He was now as sure as ever that the babies were joined at the abdomen, and almost as sure that they shared at least a liver. I knew why he believed this, as I had watched him tune-in flow coloration on the ultrasound screen. It certainly seemed as though there was some sort of flow from one baby to the other across the area at which they were joined. We were hoping that this might be the umbilical cord, and mentioned the same to the doctor. He said it might possibly be the cord, but did not sound too excited about the idea. We were still hoping and praying that the babies were not, or at least only slightly, joined. The thought that they might share vital organs, however, began creeping into our minds.

Doctor Pielet and the staff at Lutheran General are knowledgeable and competent professionals. Their areas of expertise, however, are prenatal and neonatal care. Doctor Pielet made it clear to us from the beginning, that separation surgery would have to be performed where appropriate experts were readily available. This, most likely, would be out of state. The time had come for us to begin looking for the right facility and the right doctors to perform the delicate surgery. In this area, Doctor Pielet was a great help. He had done some research, and made contact with at least three separate doctors, each of which had performed separation surgery on several previous occasions. It began to look as though we would have to make arrangements out of state, probably California or Washington DC. Sandi and I began trying to figure out which would work best. I had relatives in California, but I hadn't seen them for a while. Washington might be better, as we had already heard of an organization that would help find us a place to stay during surgery and recovery. In the long run, we agreed, we would go wherever it was best for the babies.

One of the surprises Doctor Pielet had received, was to find out from a prominent colleague, that the former chief surgeon at Children's Memorial here in Chicago, had performed several such procedures himself. We wondered why, with all that was in the news recently, we hadn't heard about any such operations being performed at Children's. The answer to this question seemed to make sense.

This doctor just had no use for the media. He refused to be involved with them in any way. As a matter of fact, he would not even consider performing the surgery if any reporters or cameras would be at all involved.

The issue of possible media attention had crossed my mind. Sandi and I had not, however, really talked about it before. This doctor's attitude, we agreed, was fine with us. We wanted to know at what point we would need to approach him. Doctor Pielet explained that he would be happy to set up the initial contact for us if we agreed, but he cautioned that this would not happen until later in the pregnancy. The reason was pretty simple.

Any doctor who considered performing such surgery, would need to have all the details of the pregnancy, including how the babies were joined, and what organs they may share and/or lack. There were still a number of weeks and several tests left before we would have gathered all the data we possibly could.

In the midst of all that was happening, Sandi and I were attempting to lead otherwise normal lives. We had planned a Thanksgiving week trip to Florida to see Sandi's parents and take in Disney World. We went ahead with our plans, driving there and back during Sandi's fourth month of pregnancy. It was a worthwhile trip, and certainly took a lot of the emotional pressure away for a while. Just being out the of area and away from all of the well meaning questions gave us the opportunity to clear our minds a little, and get ready for the more difficult times ahead.

In Florida we kept quite busy, seeing as many of the sights as possible, while still spending quality time with Sandi's family. We made sure to take care of our spiritual needs as well. In fact, we not only attended Mass, but also took in the Sunday service with Sandi's parents. They were proud to introduce us to their church community, and we knew we could use the opportunity to say a few more prayers for our babies.

Getting back to Illinois and more regular activities meant finishing some of the pre-birth duties we had been ignoring, and continuing the evaluation of our twins.

I mentioned earlier that Sandi and I had been trying for a son. Once the pregnancy got complicated, it didn't seem to matter all that much anymore. We just wanted healthy babies. Of course, we were curious as to the sex of the twins. Normally, an ultrasound at 15 weeks is fairly conclusive in this matter. Quite a while before then, we were pretty sure what we were having. For some unknown or unpublished reason, most conjoined twins are female. I believe it probably has something to do with the fact that, as they say, the female is the better survivor. In any case, the statistics said approximately 70 to 80% were girls. Based on the information we had seen, however, it was more like 80 to 90%.

One of the tests which had been performed in conjunction with a standard ultrasound, was the amniocentesis.

This was performed mainly to verify that the twins did not suffer from any genetic disorders. It would also verify the sex of the babies, and give the doctors some idea of just how developed the lungs were. To begin with, the doctor had to draw fluid from the amniotic sac, without touching either baby. The ultrasound was used to help guide the needle.

I wasn't able to be present for the first amnio, so Terry, one of our friends, went with Sandi. To make sure I wouldn't miss anything, they videotaped it. Unfortunately, although interesting to me, it was not very pleasant for Sandi. She had a very large hypodermic stuck in her tender belly, and had to remain perfectly still in order to reduce the risk of permanent damage to one of the babies. To make matters worse, before Doctor Pielet could draw any significant amount of fluid, her uterus collapsed. He was forced to withdraw and begin again. Sandi was not happy with the process.

Three weeks later, however, when the doctor notified us of the results, the pain of the amnio was, at least temporarily, forgotten. "Except for being joined, the babies appear to be 'normal' and healthy," he said. The test had, incidentally, verified the sex of the twins. They were indeed girls. We were pleased with the results. Although we knew it wasn't possible, we wished that this test could have also, somehow, helped to identify just what was inside each of our babies.

I'm sure it's not necessary to explain why it was so important to identify organs and other internals. There are certain ones a baby must have to survive at all. There are others which must be present in order to allow the child to function physically in any way close to normal. The absence or reduction of a bowel, for instance, might mean anything from a somewhat routine colostomy, to a life of bedridden intravenous feeding. The blunt truth was that either or both of our girls could end up anywhere from almost complete and fully functional to just a memory. It brought a tear to my eye then, and still does today.

The ultrasound tests which they continued to perform, were indirectly helping to identify shared tissue and organs. As part of the examination, the doctor and technician were searching each twin (now referred to as A and B) to find which organs were present. By identifying various organs, and their location in each baby, they were eliminating negative possibilities regarding those particular organs. Organ by organ the prognosis was improving.

We were beginning to get used to the emotional ups and downs between visits to the doctor. It became a little easier to answer questions and talk about our daughters. We had become even more determined that this story would end up a happy one, and thus decided to finish the pleasant task of naming our babies.

Fanning is originally an Irish name. We thought it might be nice to give our girls names that would reflect that portion of their heritage. We chose Shannon, which is Gaelic although not used in Ireland, and means "small but Wise", for one name. This we gave to the more active of the two; the twin that seemed to get Sandi's attention with rapid kicks each time something she didn't like happened. The less active but larger twin we called Megan. This name is used throughout the British Isles, and means "the strong one." Her size and disposition seemed to indicate the name was appropriate. In any case, our girls would now be known by more than "Twin A" and "Twin B."

Doctor Pielet had set up an MRI (Magnetic Resonance Imaging) exam to take place just after New Years (Jan. 5). We were hoping that this would give us some additional data to help determine just what was connected, what was shared and, God forbid, what was missing. It was a long process, with hundreds of images being generated.

In order to get clear pictures, it was necessary to make sure the babies did not move for several hours. To accomplish this, a paralyzing drug was used. This was a scary procedure to begin with, but to make matters worse, the shots were administered through Sandi's stomach, the same as for an amnio. Also, because the drug tended to follow the blood circulation from one baby to the other, they gave a double dose to the poor twin who just happened to have her bottom side stuck up toward mom's belly.

Unfortunately, these test results were, for the most part, inconclusive.

The doctors had told us that the drug should wear off in two to three hours. We began to worry when it had been more than five hours I know how I felt, and I can only imagine what Sandi was thinking that night when, ten hours had passed, and the babies were still motionless. She prayed silently that they would awaken soon. Then, after twelve hours, they began to move. They were alive and well.

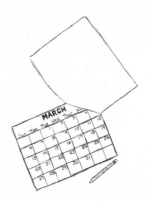

CHAPTER 4

Solid Planning

New Years had come and gone, it was a bitterly cold week, and we were planning. Doctor Pielet had already told Sandi that she would most likely have to go on bed rest sometime in January. On January 12th, he confirmed this and ordered her not to return to work. Since she worked in my department, we made plans for covering duties while she was away. The doctor expected this to be for about six months.

Other planning continued as well. We had engaged, by this time, in several discussions on the possible locations and/or doctors for the separation. The recent case which had received so much publicity involved the Lakeberg family from Indiana.

The mother had given birth to twin girls who shared a heart. We talked a little about this case with our doctors. As it turned out, the Lakeberg twins were separated in Philadelphia. Word had it that the decision was partially a financial one, and partially a political one. Apparently,

Loyola Hospital, and possibly others in our own area, had refused to perform the surgery for ethical and/or medical reasons. Sandi and I didn't really want to talk much about the Lakebergs. Their story had been a sad one, with some negative side issues. We felt ours was a happy one. Whatever outside issues might arise would only be positive.

Further discussions had taken place with the surgeons at Children's Memorial. Based on what they had seen so far, the separation surgery could be performed at their facility. Doctor Pielet had also reviewed the case with Doctor O'Neal in Philadelphia. He agreed that Children's could handle the case, and offered his services if we felt it necessary. At this time of course, we were still unsure of just what was shared. Sandi and I decided to speak with the surgeon from Children's before making any sort of decision. We also, of course, wanted to check him out. Doctor Pielet said he would call Doctor Raffensperger at Children's whenever we were ready to talk.

Everything we had heard about Raffensperger, medically and ethically, was very good. It was said he had been involved in separating at least three other sets of conjoined twins. It began to look as though our decision might be an easy one. We would meet with Children's Memorial surgeons in the near future.

In the meantime, our knowledge on the subject of conjoined twins continued to increase. There was another TV special about "Siamese" twins. This was a particularly touching story of twin girls born in Ireland and separated several years later in England. The girls were beautiful, but were joined more severely than our daughters seemed to be.

42

We watched it primarily to see what information, medical or otherwise, we could obtain. It turned out, however, to have such an emotional effect on me, that any technical information was, initially lost. Luckily, though, we did videotape it.

I noticed while reviewing the tape, two items that concerned me deeply. First of all, even with all the organs and anatomical parts that were shared or missing, the doctors were, surprisingly, most concerned about the liver(s). Secondly, one of the doctors stated that the chances of survival for conjoined twins increase by 90% , when surgery is performed after they are no longer in the infant stage. I almost wished I had not watched the special. It certainly seemed like we were fighting the odds with our little girls.

I could only take comfort in the fact that, even with all the cases we had read about and seen, there still had been no twins joined the same as our little ones. I decided it might be best, at that time, not to talk to Sandi about my added concerns after watching the tape. She was still very positive about everything, and I didn't want to do anything to change that. I knew it was also possible that she had noticed these same things during the initial broadcast, and was similarly trying to spare me.

Late in January, we received an unusual opportunity to, as we thought, increase our knowledge of conjoined twins even more. Doctor Flannery called Sandi to let her know that there was going to be a Bioethics symposium on conjoined twins at Edward Hospital in Naperville. Since it was to take place during my regular working hours, it would be very difficult for me to attend. Sandi, however, seemed well enough to violate the bed rest dictated by Doctor Pielet for two or three hours. Meghan said she would keep a close eye on her and not let her get excited.

I'm sure that since the notice of the symposium was only sent to those in the medical field, the speaker anticipated that the audience would be composed of the same. In fact, Sandi and her friend Terry, were apparently the only non-medical field associates there. This gave them a rather uncensored, unbiased look at the presentation.

As it turned out, the speaker seemed to focus on the moral and financial issues involved in the care and separation of conjoined twins; and, more specifically on the Lakeberg case. Interestingly enough, he had initially been rather closely involved. He certainly seemed to have a generally unfavorable attitude toward the Lakebergs' and any similar situation. There was, however, some knowledge to be gained. We got a good idea of just how costly separation and related care could be; and, the good doctor also explained the ethical problems involved in this specific case.

After the symposium, Meghan and Sandi approached the doctor for some further questioning. He was apparently a bit shaken when he was told that Sandi was carrying conjoined twins. He hadn't expected this from one of the attendees. He did regain his composure, and offer to provide assistance in whatever way he could. Sandi wasn't really impressed. She had taken enough notes, and we would discuss it all that evening.

As it turned out, there wasn't a whole lot to talk about. I

was rather surprised to learn that such a large amount of the total cost involved in the Lakeberg case was unpaid. I was also disturbed to hear that some medical people felt the Lakeberg couple may have continued the with pregnancy and separation for all the wrong reasons. We had discussed the issue of cost only briefly. It didn't seem to be that important with all of the other issues involved. We had insurance. We knew it wouldn't cover everything, but there were many more important things to be concerned with. Every case was different, and there were just too many undetermined issues right now. I was sure we would discuss it further at some later date.

By the time Sandi was entering her fifth month, I had used up most of my available personal time at work. This meant it was becoming very difficult for me to go along for every check-up. We decided that I should go only when we deemed it to be truly necessary. In other words, if a major test was planned, or an important decision was required.

Our visits to Lutheran General continued to include full ultrasound examinations as well as the normal pregnancy checks and measures. During one of the ultrasound exams, the technician asked if we wanted to know the sex of each baby. We both smiled a bit and said sure. "Well", she said, "this one's a girl, let's see about the other." Of course it shouldn't take a genius to know that if they're joined, they're identical. The tech realized this after she saw us both laughing. "Now that would really be one for the records," Sandi said. "A girl and a boy conjoined!"

The examinations also included some conversation regarding either steps which we might take to determine how severely the twins were joined, or when and where separation would take place. There was now very little doubt they were joined. The continuing positioning of each twin, the way one reacted in regards to movement by the other, and the apparent flow of blood indicated on the ultrasounds made it pretty clear.

Through the weeks that passed, our emotions were not all that were experiencing unusual and/or sudden changes. Sandi had, almost from the beginning of the pregnancy, felt "different." She had never carried twins before, so she wasn't really sure how she should expect to feel. Still, she seemed to be having a more difficult time than might be expected. There were hurts and pains in areas where she had never experienced such in the past.

We talked about it at some length, wondering if, because the twins were joined, they could not turn in a manner which would allow them both sufficient room. This seemed logical, and might have explained some of it, but certainly not all. We also surmised that some of it might simply be the result of the changes her body was quickly undergoing out of necessity. Whatever the reasons, she was quite uncomfortable most all of the time.

Along with the other hurts she was experiencing, Sandi was also having what seemed to be labor pains. Of course it was much too early for safe delivery of the twins. In earlier conversations held with the doctors at Lutheran General, it was mentioned that, with proper pre-natal care, successful delivery could take place after only twenty-five weeks of gestation. Doctor Pielet had, however, cautioned us that such success would be extremely unlikely given the particular problems existing with this pregnancy. He contended that we needed at least 34 weeks gestation. Anything less would put both babies (even in the most positive scenario) in extreme danger. Sandi needed to take it easier, and stay completely off her feet. She agreed with the doctor, and promised she would do all required to give our babies the best chance.

The drive from Naperville to Lutheran General is a fairly long one, taking 50 minutes in a non-rush hour situation. A lot of things can happen in that time. Labor pains could start up again. A doctor can stop labor. If it has been going on for fifty minutes or more, however, it becomes a lot more difficult.

Doctor Pielet wasn't going to take anymore chances. On February 22nd, Sandi showed up for her scheduled appointment. It turned out to be a long visit. Doctor Pielet was not going to let her go home. The examination showed that she had already partially dilated. For the next four and one half weeks, she would be confined to the hospital, and most often, to her bed as well.

Up to this point, I have not mentioned Tanja. Tanja Wagner was, at that time, our Au Pair; or, as sometimes jokingly referred to, our "mean German Au Pair." She was in the United States (legally) for one year, to provide in-home child care. She was extremely helpful and very understanding throughout this episode of our lives.

Tanja had accompanied Sandi on that final visit to Lutheran General. She brought her car home, along with some specific instructions and Sandi's youngest daughter. It appeared, at the time, that my wife anticipated Doctor

Pielet's move; although she did not agree with it.

With Sandi in the hospital, it got just a little more crazy. There were a lot of things we needed to do together, and now we would be apart more often than not. I was quite busy at work, and had two step daughters at home to take care of. In addition, Lutheran General was a hefty drive from Naperville, and the weather had turned bad. As a matter of fact, it snowed the first day she was there. The roads were pretty bad, and we didn't feel it would be a good idea to try and make the long drive with two young children. After that, I wasn't sure just how often I would be seeing Sandi. Planning would be more difficult now, just at a time when we were going to have to make some important decisions.

I knew my wife well enough to realize she would be very unhappy if not allowed to perform some important duties. Sure enough, one of the first things she wanted to tell me was that she would need me to bring her all of our mail, so that she could pay the bills and otherwise correspond as necessary. I must say that I was not one of those husbands who would turn total financial control of their life over to their wife. I had quite successfully managed my own finances for a good period of time. In truth, however, Sandi had been managing our checkbook since we were married, although I performed periodic spot-checks as I felt appropriate. Having her handle the finances now would certainly make some things easier for me. As it turned out, we more or less compromised. I performed whatever financial duties we felt made sense, and she took care of the rest from her bed. It gave her something to do, other than cross stitch.

I will say that, although I missed her at home, having Sandi in the hospital certainly lightened some of the medical concerns I had. She was right there where they could monitor her and react quickly to anything which might happen; and what did happen more often than not, was labor. The twins were really trying to come very early, much too early! A combination of specific drugs, monitoring and physical restrictions, seemed to hold them back for now. I kept wondering, though, how long it would be until the contractions became unstoppable.

Would some other complication also come into the picture? The doctors were obviously doing their best to eliminate any such situations, but there was just no way anyone could know for sure.

The question of the two babies getting entangled in one and others' cords did not seem to be an issue with our twins. So far, the ultrasounds had failed to identify separate cords. As a matter of fact, the specific identification of one single cord had not been very positive. Sandi had been at least partially correct. Being joined did eliminate one of the risks involved with twins in the same sack.

During Sandi's stay in the hospital, much more discussion took place regarding planning. Doctor Pielet was still very concerned about the possibility that the twins might be born prior to the 34th week of gestation. He continued close monitoring, and prescribed each and every precaution he believed might help reach the magic number. In the meantime, we talked more about what to expect to see when the twins were born.

A time was set up for us to visit the neonatal intensive care unit at the hospital. Since our babies would almost certainly be premature, they wanted us to know what to expect. It was an interesting experience.

The unit contained babies which had been delivered anywhere from twenty-five weeks to approximately thirty-six weeks gestation. Some of them were doing very well; others, sadly, not well at all. All of them had some sort of equipment attached. This varied from simple respirator devices to IVs, to heat lamps, and so on. The tour was not really uplifting to begin with. Once we were there for a few minutes, however, and got to see how much love and care was given to each and every child, we felt much better.

They showed us where they would be setting aside a special area for the girls, so as to draw as little unnecessary attention as possible. The rules for entry into the NICU were strictly enforced, the doctors just thought it would be better to limit the amount of attention paid to the twins by other parents, visitors and medical staff. We appreciated their feelings. Sandi and I left the unit feeling satisfied that our babies would be cared for and loved, however long their stay.

The more discussions we had, the more it became evident that we were really going to be facing two major events. The first being a successful birth; the second the undoubtedly difficult separation surgery. Doctor Pielet and the staff had been doing everything possible to get us all through the first event. It was time to start concentrating more on the second. We would set up an appointment with Doctor Raffensperger as soon as was convenient.

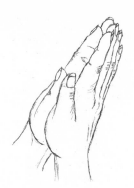

CHAPTER 5

The Art of Waiting

Preparation is perhaps the smallest, but almost certainly the most important element of waiting.

In our case there was one much larger portion. That element we call prayer. My eyes still moisten every time I recall the friends, family members and acquaintances who offered prayers for our unborn twins. Maybe in a way this was also a part of the preparation. In any case, we can never say enough about the part such prayer played in our story.

Sandi and I prayed together for the lives of our unborn children. We prayed separately for the strength and understanding to make correct decisions and accept what God had in store for us. One of the things I prayed for was the ability to choose the best doctors and/or the best hospital to perform the separation. We had heard some stories about why some institutions and some doctors might want to be involved. We did not want anyone performing such critical surgery on our children just for the experience. They had to know what they were doing, and be doing it for the right reason. I would have a lot of questions for Doctor Raffensperger, and I knew Sandi would as well.

Doctor Pielet set up the meeting for us. The doctors agreed that, since Sandi was residing at Lutheran General for a while, it would be handiest just to meet there. A date was set, and the hospital reserved a conference room for us. Doctor Raffensperger was told we would have questions for him. He had expected this would be the case. Sandi and I had been working separately on lists of questions. The week before the meeting we went over our lists together. Strangely enough, we each had 15 questions. I laughed when I read her list. "This is like reading my own list", I said. "You have only one question not on my list, and I have only one question not on yours." We had both expected that might be the case. It seemed as though we thought too much alike for any other outcome.

Doctor Pielet had informed us that there would be two doctors from Children's meeting with us that day. The first, we knew, would be Raffensperger, the second would be a close associate of his. I must admit, I was a little worried at first. I guess I had some doubts as to whether or not I would be able to tell if these were the right surgeons. After all, we were placing our daughters' very lives in their hands.

The day of our meeting, however, I felt much more confident. We had a long list of questions and I knew what answers we wanted to hear. Something else was happening as well. I was beginning to understand just how special the twins really were. It's not that they were better than anyone else. It wasn't that kind of special. It was more like I was finally seeing how wonderful the miracle of life is, and how special it was that so many people cared enough and could do enough to help our daughters experience this miracle.

Doctor Raffensperger turned out to be very much as we had expected. He was experienced, knowledgeable and professional. Some of the time he appeared to be very understanding, while at other times, he was quite blunt. He introduced himself and his associate, Doctor Luck, who seemed to be a few years younger than him, and was quite content to let him do the majority of the talking. She came across, none-the-less, as competent and understanding.

They began by asking some basic questions about Sandi's health, and the general condition of the babies. This served to break the ice and get the meeting moving. Doctor Raffensperger mentioned the list of questions we had prepared, and asked us to go through them one at a time. Sandi and I shared the duty, each asking several. For the most part, their answers were direct and complete. It appeared they really knew their stuff. They went on to answer most of our remaining questions, and then began explaining how separation would take place.

It sounded pretty simple when I first heard it. There would be 2 operating teams and 2 operating tables. As soon as separation occurred, one twin would be taken to the other table for whatever additional surgery might be necessary. When he went into more detail on the initial surgery, however, it became clear that it was to be far from simple. There were a number of unknowns which would have to be clarified before the direction or extent of the surgery could be determined.

The doctors next talked about the current prognosis for the babies. Along with this, they gave us some explanations of what each possibility might represent. At this point it began to get a little scary.

"You're both engineers," said Doctor Raffensperger, "and I'm not, but I'm going to draw you a picture anyway."

I remember thinking how his drawing resembled the outline of one of those ink blots. You know the ones you're supposed to look at and tell somebody what you see. It didn't look much like our daughters, that was for sure. It turned out that the picture he drew represented the liver (or livers) the girls shared.

"This is what we feel the situation is," he said. "The babies seem to be joined at the livers or sharing a single liver. Hopefully we will be able to tell more after they are born, and we get a chance to run some additional tests. We are unsure yet, as to what else they may share, and to what extent. It looks right now as if there may be some bowel in here as well. Doctor Pielet seems to feel that is the case. It's going to be pretty important to know what the situation is for sure. We may not be able to tell, however, until after the surgery begins. We have to be prepared for whatever different possibilities may exist. If it turns out there is bowel involved, it could mean several different things. Let me explain to you what the three basic possibilities are concerning how severely they are joined."

"First of all, they may only be joined by some muscle tissue and a portion of each liver. If this is the case, separation is pretty simple. I could teach a school kid to do it. You just make a cut basically right down the middle."

"The second possibility is that the babies either share a liver, or have two livers growing together, and also share some bowel or other organ which can be divided. If this is the case, there are a number of additional possibilities, depending, for instance, on how much bowel and how it is shared. As long as both babies have a rectum, we can cut where the bowel is joined, give some to each baby then reattach the ends. Should one baby be missing a rectum, however, the outlook would be very grim."

"The third possibility is that one baby is missing a vital organ or has some other extremely severe abnormality. If this turns out to be the case, there will be little or no hope of saving that child. Our position in cases like this has been to do everything possible for the twin having the best chance. This is an issue we must get your agreement on in advance. From what I have seen, however, it appears as though we are looking at some version of the second possibility."

Up until this time, we had believed that a liver could easily be successfully divided. All of the knowledgeable medical people had basically told us that "if they're going to share an organ, the liver is the best one." Some of them had explained how the remaining portion of the liver would actually regenerate to a size appropriate to the particular individual. One even mentioned a recent case in which a portion of a child's liver was removed and surgically attached in place of the failing liver in his own mother. Both parent and child were healthy and doing well.

One thing they failed to mention, however, was that in order to function, the liver must have a bile duct. When Doctor Raffensperger explained this to us, we both became very quiet. All these weeks we had been thinking that if they only shared a liver, the surgery would not be as difficult, and the girls would quite possibly be fully functional afterwards.

The doctor went on to explain in a little more detail. The whole thing, unfortunately, made sense. You could cut off a portion of a healthy liver and transplant it successfully, because normally the recipient would have her own liver. The bile duct would still be there and intact. "We have been unable to successfully construct an artificial bile duct. The best one I know of worked for only a short while. If the twins have only one duct, the outcome for one of the babies would be very grim indeed."

We knew of course what he meant. Even as he went on speaking, I silently prayed that the second duct would be there. Doctor Raffensperger continued explaining various aspects of the surgery, and what to expect. It was difficult to focus clearly on what he was saying all of the time, with the issue of the bile duct clouding our minds. Eventually, however, we managed to bring our full attention back to the current subject.

The doctor was discussing the issue of decisions in the operating room. "When we're in surgery, the main goal of everyone there will be to keep both babies alive. No one dies in the operating room. There are decisions, however, which may need to be made on an immediate basis."

I don't remember the exact wording he used from this point on, but the meaning was clear. What he said was basically that they did not believe in putting the healthy child at high risk in order to sustain the other child, if that other child had no chance at a quality life. Again, here was some aspect of the whole ordeal we had not really thought about. It was now necessary, however, for us to understand the philosophy involved, and the considerations to be taken into account. I remember thinking at the time how ridiculous the term "normal conjoined pregnancy" seemed. It was a real oxymoron.

The conversation then moved on to some of the lighter details. We talked about the total number of medical people to be involved, the approximate time duration, and the subsequent recovery period. Doctor Raffensperger said there would be two surgical teams, with five to eight people on each. If things went well and there were no surprises, the surgery could be completed in as little as three hours. If there were unforeseen circumstances or difficulties, however, it might last eight hours or more. The recovery period was hard to predict until we knew the extent of the required surgery. The best guess was that they would need to be in the hospital anywhere from several weeks to several months.

One of the questions on both our lists was: When will the surgery take place? We had previously believed it might take place anywhere from a few days after birth to a number of months after. We were really hoping it would be very soon after the delivery. The thought of trying to move the girls around and keep them safe and comfortable while they were joined, really concerned us. As Sandi had mentioned earlier "I've never seen conjoined car seats." It was true! There would be a real challenge in just taking them home from the hospital.

The doctor was quite helpful in this matter. "We would like to operate as soon as possible after delivery," he said. "We would wait until they had been stabilized here at Lutheran General, and were doing fine. Then we would want to run some tests prior to the surgery. That should take two to three days. The surgery would begin directly following, unless something showed up which gave us a reason to wait."

This made us feel a lot better. The twins would not be going home at all prior to surgery. There would be no need for special clothing, car seat, etc. There was, however, another reason for concern. Sandi would be having the babies by cesarean section. Doctor Pielet had already said he would need a lot of room to get them out safely. How likely would it be that he would release her from the hospital only three days after such surgery? If she were not released, then the twins would be at another hospital an hour's drive away; and I would be with them. She would be stuck here alone, away from her newborns, while they were undergoing critical surgery.

We knew enough to realize that one or both of their lives might well be in grave danger at that time. Emotionally, this would be extremely difficult for Sandi. We would need to talk about this after the meeting.

Two of the last questions we had prepared for the doctors, did not involve any medical issues. We wanted to know it they would be taking any pictures or film of the procedure. We also wanted to know if they would allow anyone else to do the same. They stated that they may have some photos taken for medical purposes, but they definitely would not allow videotaping.

At this point, Doctor Raffensperger seemed to show a bit of concern. "Does the media know about this?" he asked. "No", I said. "We have not told anyone. We just wanted to know what your policy is regarding this issue." He went on to explain the problems he saw with having the news media involved. "They tend to make a circus of everything. They get in the way and they put their equipment in the way. You must also remember, as I said before, everyone in the operating room will be doing their best to keep both babies alive. A nurse, technician or other doctor may disagree with a doctors split second decision. This may be only temporary, but if the media is there, they will blow it out of proportion."

He didn't ask why we wanted to know about the media, but we thought it was probably pretty clear. We had finally come to realize that there would, at least initially, be a lot of interest in the twins. That is, of course if someone were to let the word out. Knowing how much the Lakebergs were in the news, we could assume the Fannings would be there almost as much. We were trying to protect our privacy and our own personal interests. If there were to be film and/or photos, we wanted control over them.

He concluded talk on the subject by saying: "The hospital may be taking some stills of the procedure." By the way he had addressed the whole issue, we sensed that what others had told us was true. He had little use and no love for the media, and would likely not perform the operation if they were involved.

Before concluding the meeting, we went over a lot of the simple details like: check-in, approval signatures, and hospital contacts. We concluded with both doctors giving us their card and phone number so that we could call if we came up with additional questions or concerns.

After the meeting, Sandi and I discussed what had occurred. These doctors really seemed to know their stuff. We believed them to be honest, professional and caring. Their plan of procedure appeared to be just what was required. It was neither too elaborate, nor too simple. As long as Doctor Pielet agreed, and no additional negative discoveries took place, the babies were going to Children's Memorial.

We also discussed the possibility of Sandi having to remain at Lutheran General, while Megan and Shannon were undergoing surgery at Children's. Sandi didn't see a real problem, as doctor Pielet had assured her he would let her leave as soon as she was able to stand. Everyone was sure that Children's would supply a wheelchair for her if necessary. She felt three days would be more than enough time for her to get back on her feet. I hoped she was right. Having us miles apart at such a time would make things tremendously difficult.

It felt good to get that decision out of the way. I really wished that a lot more of the unknowns could be answered just by us making decisions. Those decisions, however, were to be made by someone much higher up.

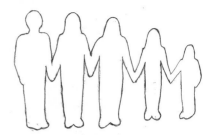

CHAPTER 6

Preparing The Family

It seems that everyone loves a newborn baby. The fresh innocence, the need for tender loving care, even the helpless cry, all add to the wonder we experience when a child first enters the world.

We wanted our twins to generate those same feelings. Was this going to be possible? As far as we were concerned, it sure was. Sandi and I wanted the rest of our family to see the babies as soon as possible, and to share the love and wonder we knew we would experience. We believed in our hearts, that the twins' brother and sisters would not see the them as being "different" or in any way frightening.

They had already assured us, at Lutheran General, that our other children would get a chance to see the girls before they were transferred to Children's.

This was very important to us. We had to be realistic, and admit that there was a possibility they may not be able to see both girls after the separation surgery. Sandi and I also thought it would be best if the other kids got a good look at conjoined twins before surgery. This would help them to both understand what Megan and Shannon would be going through, and to see that there was nothing terrible or "freaky" about the twins.

For Sandi's daughters it was a fairly simple issue. Amanda was eight years old, and Rachel four. They would accept whatever we told them. Even if they didn't agree, they would not give us too hard of a time. Besides, they missed mom and wanted to see her regardless of the circumstances. They were also pretty excited about getting two new sisters. Seeing the twins while they were at the hospital to visit mom, would be sort of a lucky coincidence.

The story was different with my three children. They were all adults living away from home, although Paul did stay at home during college break. Laura and Leanne had both been very supportive of us. They had been concerned about the problems in the pregnancy from the beginning, and were now anxious and positive about seeing their little sisters. We knew they would want to be there.

Besides having lives of their own, however, they regularly saw their mother. It was necessary to consider her feelings as well. She had not accepted my remarrying very well. She might be a little hurt if they showed very much attention to my new family. I certainly did not envy the position any of them was in. I did know them well enough, however, to believe that they would at least consider my request to have them present.

As it turned out, they all made me quite proud. They read the situation very well, and agreed to come see the twins as soon as possible after birth. My daughters were quite surprised that their brother had agreed to be there. He had, for some time, stayed away from any and all births, deaths, weddings, funerals, birthdays and holiday celebrations. It wasn't necessarily that he didn't like us, or did not consider us as his family. It was just Paul's way based on what he believed in. He had changed during the last few years. Having always been an idealistic youth, he had now grown critical of many of the traditions connected with "the institution."

Readily agreeing to be present at the birth did not seem like his style, which made me even happier.

As for the other members of our family, they all knew that the babies were joined; and they had some general knowledge of the dangers ahead. Most of them also voiced desires to see the twins as soon as they possibly could. A good number lived out of state, which would make it very difficult in any case.

Sandi's immediate family consisted of her two parents and one sister. All of whom lived in Florida. She had a grandmother, an aunt and uncle, and various other relatives who lived either here in Illinois, or out of state. My family was a bit larger. I had four brothers, seven sisters and a mother living in various states and in Canada. I also had aunts and uncles on both sides of my family as well as more cousins, nephews and nieces than I could remember. A good number of them did live in the Chicago area, but many more were out of state.

Sandi's parents were already making plans to come to Illinois that spring. My mother lived in Colorado with two of my sisters. She was no longer capable of making such long trips by automobile, and would not fly for any reason.

We really didn't mind. Having the twins in all of the family's thoughts and prayers was as good as, or better than, having them all at the hospital with us. We hoped there would be lots of time and many opportunities for them to meet the rest of the family later on.

Sandi and I had agreed early on that only the necessary people should know about the girls being conjoined. Those who knew the most were the immediate family members. In the case of my three sisters living in Illinois, this included their children.

There were a number of relatives who had problems of their own. There was no need to add ours to their piles. This group included Sandi's grandmother and one of my aunts who had been extremely close to my mother, as well as others. Of course, as I mentioned earlier, there were a number of friends and co-workers who also knew anywhere from the basics, to some finer details of the situation. It's rather difficult to see people every day, have them ask about the pregnancy, know they are concerned and yet keep them in the dark. From all of these people, we expected the same thing. That they should respect our privacy, keep what they had been told confidential and understand our reasons for wanting it that way.

The fact that no one representing any radio or television station, or any news periodical had called us or either hospital about the twins, led us to believe that our trust in all of these people was well-founded.

The question of the media and possible involvement did come up in conversations with some family members. Our position was always about the same. We were not going to let anyone make a circus out of this, or make the girls out to be "unusual" in any way. We had seen and heard a lot of unpleasant things regarding some similar cases. Ours was going to be different, and much more positive. We were going to do our best to make sure it stayed that way.

Still, when Sandi and I talked privately, we realized that sooner or later something should be said. After the Lakeberg case had generated so much sadness, it would be nice to see something really positive and happy about conjoined twins.

We reached an agreement. After surgery was successfully completed, and it was no longer possible for reporters and/or cameras to interfere, we would have someone contact one of the television stations. That way, only accurate information would be passed on to the news media. Everyone would know that we had cooperated. And yet, no one would be in a position to have any effect on the critical decisions we would be making. It would be too late for interference.

I had never really dealt with the news media, but from what I had seen and heard, we would need to be prepared for some personal and possibly ill-timed questions. I did not want Sandi to have to deal with that issue while so many other things were still in question. We would hold any further conversation off until the time and circumstances were more appropriate.

While we had no clear plan for telling all of our remaining friends and relatives about the twins, we certainly had intended to do it sooner or later. It just didn't seem all that important that they know before the surgery. We had already notified enough people that we were sure the girls were being prayed for multiple times every single day, and we were by no means looking for sympathy. It hadn't dawned on us that informing the media at the appropriate time, might guarantee that virtually everyone we had ever met would know about the girls within hours.

I continued to answer questions from friends and relatives about Sandi and the pregnancy. It seemed everyone at work wanted to know how she was doing as well, and what the latest prognosis was. I was as gracious as I could be, and told them as much as I thought appropriate. It wasn't easy, however. The questions always got me thinking about the upcoming birth. Although I managed to maintain my position of hope and faith in the future. I could not filter out all the negative images which worked their way into these thoughts. The odds against the twins ever being completely "normal" were very great. As a matter of fact, unless everything went perfectly from this point on, the odds against both of the twins surviving were high. No matter how confident I managed to appear on the outside, I knew somewhere inside, that only a real miracle would make the story of our twins a truly happy one.

Sandi, on the other hand, had phone calls and questions of her own to answer. A number of people were calling her once a day for updates. She seemed to take it all very well. Each time I visited, I found her to be in good spirits and a positive frame of mind. She wasn't going to let any negative thoughts crowd her plans for these two children.

Because Sandi was so positive, and we both kept our happy faces on, some people actually doubted the seriousness of the situation. I guess they expected us to go around with long faces every day and complain to anyone who would listen. That mode of behavior was far from our minds. We believed that we could really help get positive results by having positive attitudes. I believe that's why some of these same people were to comment, months later, on how well we handled ourselves and what a good job we did of covering up the potential problems.

The truth was, however, regardless of how it seemed, outwardly, I was extremely worried and sometimes maybe even scared.

Had the ultrasound examinations, and other tests shown what we hoped for, there would not have been as much reason for concern. The reality was, however, as we passed the thirtieth week and headed into the final weeks of the pregnancy, we knew very little more than we had early on. The babies were almost undoubtedly joined; how severely and what organs they shared, we still did not know.

Because I was kept very busy during this period, the waiting was easier for me than for my wife. She was not able to do much of anything except wait. It had become quite uncomfortable for her when she was on her feet, and the doctors really didn't allow her out of bed much anyway. The hours for her must have been very long. I know she made everyone quite proud by handling it all so very well.

When we first realized Sandi would have to spend at least four weeks in the hospital, we knew she would have to face another issue. The doctor who had given us the original negative diagnosis was a member of the medical staff, sooner or later, he might be filling in for Doctor Pielet.

He could be examining Sandi.

She had refused to see him since our second visit, and had told Doctor Pielet she would never see him. Her reasons were clear. He had scared us terribly and hurt us deeply with his initial opinion on the twins. It was difficult to forget something which had such a huge effect on our emotions. There were just too many other things to be concerned with. The issue with this doctor needed to be resolved, and the sooner we faced it, the better we could focus on the more important issues.

During one of my earlier visits, Sandi had mentioned to me how Doctor Pielet had approached her about the other doctor. He had, apparently, explained to her that the doctor was only using the facts as he saw them to formulate and opinion. This is the way doctors must sometimes operate. At the time, Sandi said nothing in reply. She did talk about it with me, however, and we had quite a worthwhile discussion on the subject.

I had also been very upset with that doctor. I think, however, that I looked at it a little differently. From the first statement he made regarding fetal stress, I realized a comparison might exist between a doctor's prognosis and an engineer's evaluation. To come up with an decision, or a opinion, an engineer must view all of the facts, and then make a judgment based on those facts along with any experience on the subject he/she might possess. It seemed to me that, the doctor had just done the same thing.

It was easy to agree with Sandi, therefore, when she finally said she would not give anyone a hard time about seeing him. By the same token, she would not go out of her way to be accommodating either.

During the following weeks, Sandi was seen by him on several occasions. He treated her and our unborn babies with care, while showing openness and honesty. We came to see him in a different light. By the time those four and one half weeks had passed, and the twins were delivered, he had won back the respect and trust of us both.

Doctor Pielet, on the other hand, seemed to develop a bit of a sense of humor. I guess it was probably there all along, but he needed to know us better for it to show. In any case, I believe the relationship between the doctor and our family grew in warmth and sincerity as the delivery neared.

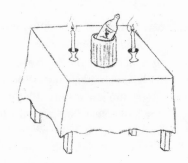

CHAPTER 7

A Miracle in Itself

Those who have witnessed the birth of their own offspring, have been indeed blessed. I will not attempt to put into words the feelings that flood over a parent during those few seconds. Suffice to say that the rest of the world seems to stand still while this miracle transpires.

I was not present for the birth of any of my first three children. In those days, many hospitals did not offer such a paternal option. My absence from the first big events of their lives did not mean that I loved them any less than I could have, or treated them any differently than I should have. It only meant that I missed three opportunities of experiencing a marvelously wonderful event first hand.

Sandi had asked me early on to be present at this birth. My reply had been quick. "I'll be there unless you really insist you don't want me to attend," I said. She smiled back and said, "Of course I want you there! You did this to me!" From then on, the only time we spoke of my presence was when the issue of video/pictures came up.

We had received an 8 mm video recorder for a wedding

gift, and I was becoming quite proficient in it's use. Actually, as long as I held and pointed it correctly, it did a good job all by itself. In any case, we really wanted someone to record the birth of the twins. It didn't have to be me, but I would do it if there was no other way. Luckily, there turned out to be someone else.

When Sandi had been in the hospital only a few days, she had an unexpected visitor. It seemed that one of my sister's sons had recently changed jobs, and was now employed by Lutheran General. My nephew Rich was an expert in media coordination. This included audio and visual taping and reproduction for the hospital.

Rich had already been up to see Sandi by the time I had found out he worked there. His being there was a bit of a blessing. Sandi now had a family member who would be able to visit her at least once a day, virtually every work day. Since the hospital was a rather long drive, visits from other relatives would be few. Most of them did make up for it by keeping her on the phone 75% of the time, but the first hand visits were the best.

Following my nephew's first visit, Sandi and I talked again about video taping the birth. As it turned out, one of the nurses Sandi had made friends with was experienced in this area, and had offered to help. Although we appreciated her offer, we both agreed that it might be better to see if Rich would do it. Sandi said she would ask him when he came by the next day.

It didn't take long for Sandi and Rich to come to an agreement on video taping. He would gladly handle it, and use our camera so that ownership of the tape would not be in question. In addition, one of Lutheran General's photographers would also be taking stills. These would belong to the hospital, but we would receive a full set of copies. Since this would still mean that all those present in the delivery room would be hospital employees, except for Sandi and I, getting full agreement was easy. All of the staff members at Lutheran General were turning out to be quite helpful and agreeable. We hoped this would help to make the delivery a little less nerve-racking. We knew, no matter what happened, it would be an extremely emotional event.

I suppose it was only natural that with the delivery becoming more and more imminent, our focus shifted somewhat away from the separation.

I say that the delivery was imminent, but at the time there were still many uncertainties. Sandi continued to experience on and off labor pains, and the hospital continued to monitor her. We still did not know how severely the girls were joined, and by the time Sandi had reached her thirtieth week, it still appeared as though the babies were not developed enough to survive on their own. It was important for everyone to remember that they were joined. The use of special life sustaining equipment would be much more difficult.

During this period of time, another concern surfaced. The doctors began to suspect that at least one of the twins had a bowel obstruction. While in the womb, this would mean very little. Once they had been born, however, it most probably would be considered life-threatening.

The doctors told us that correcting such obstructions in infants was fairly common. In the case of Megan and

Shannon, however, major surgery would be required just to get to the bowels. Of course, the obstructions could be repaired during the separation surgery, but there was still one large problem remaining. If the babies could not breathe and otherwise function on their own, the surgery could not take place. One or both would surely perish. If, however, the hospital equipment was used to keep them going until they were on their own, the bowel obstruction might kill one or both. These facts together offered us even more reasons to focus on the delivery, and to pray for the babies' rapid and complete development in their mother's womb.

At the time, I don't think we fully understood how real the danger was. We tried to remain completely positive, and as resolved as ever.

Dr. Pielet, we later realized, understood completely. He quietly and sternly demanded that we stay with the plans and steps he had prescribed. Sandi and the nurses, for instance, had brought themselves to believe that once the magic thirty weeks were achieved, Sandi might be able to come home and wait out the remaining time in the comfort of our own home, surrounded by her family. She was quite upset when, during her exam at 31 weeks, Dr. Pielet found one of the babies' feet in her cervix and refused to consider her request to leave the hospital. He feared that the tiny feet might rupture the amniotic sac or cause the cervix to dilate further. At the time everyone considered him extremely stubborn. We learned later on that his "stubbornness" was aimed strictly at saving the lives of our two babies.

During this, the most difficult portion of Sandi's hospital stay, my visits, unfortunately, did not increase. Taking additional time off from work was difficult, as I knew I would need extra time after the babies were born. To make matters worse, I was the primary person filling in for Sandi in her absence from work. I was managing to see her at least every other day, and to bring her daughters at least once a week. Sandi understood, and was satisfied to see us as often as possible. We continued, of course, to speak on the telephone numerous times each day.

There was one day, however, that I made absolutely sure I was there. This was March 7th. That day we celebrated our first wedding anniversary. It was, obviously, quite important to Sandi.

With the help of the hospital staff, who provided a private conference room, complete with video for two, I was able to bring Sandi one of her favorite dinners in celebration. The steak, lobster, baked potato and vegetable were prepared by me in advance and kept in a warmer during the drive to the hospital. For the special salad, I prepared all the ingredients ahead of time, and arranged them while Sandi was getting ready. Although she knew we would be eating together, when she saw our anniversary dinner, complete with candles, she was thrilled. I believe it really helped her get through some of the difficult times she was having.

The closer we got to the thirty-fourth week, the more questions and phone calls we received from family and friends. Their concerns were considerable and genuine. Everyone we knew seemed to have us on their minds. We were always careful to acknowledge each caller, giving only whatever update information seemed appropriate. We did not want to hurt anyone's feeling, but we also did not want everyone worrying too much about us. If I remember correctly, most of them had some sort of worries of their own. They didn't need ours. Still it was nice to know we had so much support.

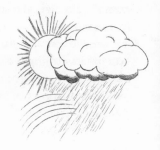

CHAPTER 8

The First Event

The week of March 20th had been a significant one. Sandi had been running an elevated temperature, and her contractions had increased. To add to the situation, she had begun discharging fluid on the 23rd. All of these things pointed to the likelihood that the babies were coming very, very soon.

All indications were, at that time, that the babies, while developing well, were not mature enough to risk the difficulties of the delivery and subsequent separation surgery. As we had already been advised, survival during separation would be unlikely, unless the vital organs were mature. This meant that, if for some reason the doctors were forced to perform the surgery shortly after birth, our twins would have little chance unless vital organs had completely matured.

The doctors decided to perform another amnio. There were two separate tests which could be performed on the amniotic fluid to help determine if the babies' lungs were mature. The first, the Fetal Lung Maturity test (FLM), was less conclusive, but could be analyzed within two hours. The second test was much more sophisticated and took a number of additional hours to process. The amnio would also be used to determine if the fluid being discharged was indeed from the amniotic sac. This would be accomplished by shooting dye into the uterus before drawing out amnio fluid. If it was amniotic fluid and/or the lungs showed up as being fully mature, the babies would be delivered the next day. Otherwise, the waiting would continue.

I was again unable to be present for the amnio. It was just as well, however, Sandi was again poked twice. When I spoke to her that evening, she was a bit apprehensive. She felt the babies were coming, one way or the other. She was hoping and praying for the lungs to test out as mature.

The results from the FLM came back about when they were expected. They were not, however, very encouraging. The readings were interpreted as indicating borderline maturity. All this did for us was give us more to worry about. If the combined reading was borderline, did that mean one baby most likely had mature lungs and the other baby almost certainly did not? The hospital could not answer that question. Everyone would just have to wait for the results of the second test.

This particular test (I don't believe we ever knew it's name) had two separate indicators. The first one was called the LS. If this reading was 2.0 or higher, it indicated mature lungs. The second reading was called the PG. This only required a reading anywhere above "zero", to indicate maturity.

It would be sometime, very early in the morning before we would know how these readings had turned out. I would go about my day as if all were normal, until I received a call from Sandi.

I went in to work as usual the morning of March 24th. It wasn't that I really wanted to be there, or that they couldn't do without me that day. The truth is, I wanted very much to be at Lutheran General. I had a real feeling that Sandi had been correct, our twins would be arriving that day. It would be necessary, however, for me to take additional time off later on, during and following the separation. I still had an obligation to the company, and wanted to let everyone know I took it seriously.

As it happened, I was in a meeting when Sandi called. Her voice gave away a mixture of emotions. I could sense joy, fear, anticipation and hope all in the few words she spoke. "They're going to take the girls!!" she said.

"When?" I asked. Realizing, of course, that she meant today. What I really wanted to know was: "How much time do I have to get everyone ready and get up there?" "Today, at 11:00 O'clock," she said. Then she went on to explain how the test results had come out. The LS reading had been at 2.2 indicating maturity. The PG reading had also indicated maturity, coming in at the .3 level. There was still a concern though. Because the twins shared amniotic fluid, the tests could not guarantee that both had mature lungs. We could still have had one with and one without.

There had been no additional leakage of fluid since the dye was inserted. Nevertheless, Sandi continued to show indications of going into full and unstoppable labor. Doctor

Pielet had no choice, they would deliver that morning. I told her I would finish things up at work and be right there. She seemed very concerned that I might be late, but I assured her I would not. "Besides," I said, "Doctor Pielet wouldn't start without me, would he." Of course he would have, but I had absolutely no intention of finding out for sure.

It was plenty early, but there were a lot of things to do and people to call. I made my apologies at the meeting and departed immediately. I knew I probably appeared more calm and cool than normal on the outside, but inside I was experiencing just about the same emotional churning as Sandi. Things were happening fast, and reality was beginning to set in.

After Sandi and I spoke, she contacted Tanja and explained what was going on. Tanja was to get Sandi's daughters ready, and take them to Lutheran General. If he planned on going at all, my son Paul would ride with them. As for Leanne and Laura, my daughters, they were ready to leave as soon as they got the call.

I placed that call before heading north to the hospital. In addition, I phoned my sister Helen. She wanted to be there for the birth, and would also pass the news on to other family members. These were but the first of literally hundreds of calls placed and received by us in the next two day period.

I got in my car and quickly headed for Lutheran General and my wife's side.

The way I felt when I first entered the hospital that day was unusual, to say the least. Let me attempt to relate this feeling to you as best I can.

Do you know how , when an event is of some significance to you, you walk around sort of expecting everyone you pass by to know about your event? It's kind of like you think they should be getting ready or something, instead of just calmly going about their business. Even worse, you might expect them to acknowledge you, as if everyone should know who you are!

Now I didn't really expect this to happen. I was just so emotionally keyed up, and my mind was racing so much, that reality seemed to be in another dimension. I was experiencing a sort of fast-forward day dream. Luckily, after a few short seconds, the racing stopped. I was back to being calm and calculating. In the whole episode, there was to be only one other time when I came close to losing control.

There would be a number of times when I would cry, or clench my fist and ask why out loud. But I would always remain in control. Tears are a physical sign of sadness, happiness, fear or frustration, but , they are not necessarily an indication of control loss. The same can be said for the release of physical or verbal anger.

I was certain then that the best way to get through this type of situation was to remain in control as much of the time as possible. I had to control myself, as the situation was, most often, beyond my control.

When I reached Sandi's floor, I began to see some familiar faces. The nurses also recognized me, and commented on how "the time was just about here." There was some good-natured joking about how I might fair through the whole event. Of course, they realized the seriousness of the situation, but had great faith in Doctor Pielet and the rest of the medical team. They were also, I was sure, trying to relax us a little. When I thought about it, I realized it was sort of nice to hear something to make me feel like a normal expectant father. It had been a long time since I had felt that way. Paul was twenty-two years old.

Sandi appeared about the same in person as she had over the phone. I gave her a big hug, and she squeezed my hand tightly. Tears welled up in her eyes as she said "our girls are coming, I know they'll be alright, but I'm just a little scared." I agreed with her that everything would be okay, and did my best to help her stay calm. Considering the circumstances, I thought she did a marvelous job herself. The past thirty weeks had been very hard on her, but she had not given up her positive attitude. She had shown inner strength and faith that no one really knew was there. I was very proud of her.

The plan for delivery of the twins was well in place. Sandi and I had spoken with the doctors about what would be happening. For the most part, it would be quite similar to any other cesarean section delivery. In our case, however, there would be some additional individuals present. They would be primarily from the neonatal group. Of course, Rich and his associate would be there taking pictures and video. One of the nurses Sandi had become friends with, Wendy, would be standing by her, taking pictures and holding her hand as required. I would be on the other side, holding her other hand and watching whatever I could of the procedure.

As I mentioned earlier, we had agreed that the babies would be moved to Children's as soon as they had been stabilized at Lutheran General. We learned that very morning, that, if everything went well, the move would take place around 1:00 P.M. the same day. It looked as though the girls would not be spending a lot of time with all the great people in the neonatal ward. We hoped the staff at Children's would be as nice.

From Sandi's hospital room, the planning continued. She wanted me to leave for Children's with the girls, so that they would not be away from at least one of us for any long period of time. The plan, on my part, was to get the babies settled in , visit with them a while, and return that evening to be with Sandi. Because of the severity of the surgical procedure required to deliver the girls, and the medication she would receive afterwards, Sandi would be in no condition to have visitors for a few hours.

My daughter Laura, her boyfriend Tom and my sister Helen would go with me to Children's. All of the other family members would return home after seeing the newborn babies.

Lutheran General had assigned a special case worker to handle our situation. Her name was Phyllis , and she was to arrange getting all of us scrubbed and ready to see the girls, two at a time. The whole thing was set up to draw as little unnecessary attention as possible to the twins.

By the time Sandi was taken to the delivery preparation area, most of the family had arrived. Helen was allowed to be in the prep room with us. I was glad to have her there. She lent Sandi strong support and, her presence made the wait more tolerable.

The family members were all there waiting together when we headed for the operating room. We took some preliminary pictures and film footage to verify the equipment was operating correctly. It also seemed to relax everyone just a little. Surprisingly enough, there really did not seem to be a lot of tension present. The air was, however, charged with a special kind of anticipation. I remember how good it made me feel, sensing so many positive vibrations. We were ready now. Our girls were coming. The wait was over.

As Sandi was prepared for the delivery, I prayed silently for God to be kind. Not necessarily to me. I hadn't really done much to deserve it, but to my wife and daughters. Sandi had done everything in her power to keep the girls healthy and strong. Megan and Shannon were innocent and helpless. Surely they deserved a chance. So many prayers had already been offered in so many different places, that I knew God was well aware of the girls' situation.

I couldn't help but recall something one of the nuns had once told us at catholic school. "God the Father is like any other parent. If you ask for something enough times, he just might give it to you so you'll stop bothering him." It sounded pretty silly right then, but I was willing to accept any idea that might improve our daughters' chances.

After some final waves and kisses, Sandi disappeared around the corner and into the delivery room. I glanced one last time at all of our family members. They seemed so excited, so willing to be a part of this birth. I have never been so proud of our children, collectively, as I was at that moment.

The operating room looked quite standard to me. As a matter of fact, seeing it along with the doctors and nurses present might have led one to believe that the upcoming delivery was to be nothing out of the ordinary; just another "c" section.

The fact that I had never seen a natural birth delivery, let alone a cesarean section, didn't make a whole lot of difference. Sandi was ready, I was ready, and we believed the girls were ready. We certainly didn't need to ask the medical team. It was easy to see they were ready also.

I'm not really the squeamish type. Nonetheless, I was sort of glad I wasn't going to get a real good look at the cutting going on. Doctor Pielet had already told us that he would need to make a very long vertical incision, and possibly a horizontal one as well. The twins would need a lot of room to come out, as they would be positioned somewhere between face-to-face and side-by-side. There was to be a curtain set up to prevent Sandi from watching the surgery. This would also prevent me from watching, unless I was to rise up from my position at her left side. (I was to take a peek a couple of times, ending up not too excited about what I had seen.) It was probably for the best that Sandi kept a tight grip on my hand, preventing me from straying too far.

In any case, it had been pre-arranged that the curtain would be dropped just as the doctors were about to actually deliver the babies. Sandi and I would both see them as they were born.

I don't know how long it was from the time the surgery actually began, to the moment the twins delivered, but it seemed to happen very quickly. One minute my mind was racing, trying to envision how they would look. The next minute the curtain was being lowered.

The entire room looked on with excitement and awe as, at 11:54 A.M., Shannon and Megan Fanning entered our world, more or less side-by-side, arms around one and other. They were so beautiful, so perfect, and both breathing on their own.

The staff quickly went about the task of cleaning the babies and otherwise preparing them for their hospital stay. Other normal delivery room activities proceeded as well. They counted limbs, toes, fingers, etc.. On the outside, at least, both girls had everything.

As might have been expected, there was only one umbilical cord; but it was large. Boy was it large, and bright blue! The color, we discovered, was due to the harmless dye which had been injected into Sandi's uterus the previous day, in order it determine if her sac was leaking. It made the cord look much more prominent than should have been the case. For those present, it was the first time they had seen such a cord. Besides being blue, it had six vessels instead of the normal three.

The first few minutes after the delivery, the room was filled with commotion. Everyone was busy taking care of the babies, operating cameras, or literally putting Sandi back together. Everyone that is, except me. I was watching it all rather awestruck.

I had seen the babies well enough to know that they were indeed joined. It seemed, however, to be more severe than what we had hoped for. The area where they were joined covered at least one third of the torso. It appeared to start just below the breast, and continued to somewhere under the area where the umbilical cord would normally have been. There was definitely more than just skin and tissue being shared. It was rather amazing though, there was nothing scary or in any way disturbing about them. They were absolutely beautiful. Even where their bodies were joined, they looked quite natural and healthy. I went over to touch my new daughters.

By this time, I was aware of the fact that Sandi was crying. I didn't have to look close to see that they were tears of joy. A quick glance also told me that at least two of the medical personnel had followed her lead. My own eyes had also become somewhat moist. I suspected that, behind their masks, others were similarly sharing the event.

After a few seconds with the girls, I went over to where the nurses were preparing the birth certificates. My purpose was twofold. I wanted to make sure they knew which baby was which, as we had named them while they were still in the womb. I also, however, wanted to make sure the time of birth was the same for both girls.

For whatever reason, some people seem to make a big deal out of which twin is born first. Sandi and I had decided that we wanted ours born at exactly the same time. This would prevent eventual problems regarding who was the older of the two. Since they were joined, simultaneous birth was only appropriate.

As it turned out, the nurse had everything correct, and only needed my input for verification.

Still a little high from having been witness to a true miracle, I went back to see my daughters. By this time, they had already been given their own little knit caps; each with a "Happy Birthday" message across the front.

The doctors, in the meantime, continued to work on Sandi. Putting her back together took a lot more time than the actual delivery. She was going to be quite sore. They had more or less filleted her uterus. Nonetheless, she insisted I go with the twins and stay with them every possible second.

The doctors had promised her that she would be able to see the girls again before they were transported. She wanted me to help make sure they kept their promise. I kissed her on the forehead and left her side.

As soon as they were ready, the twins were whisked out of the delivery room, headed for Neonatal. Just coincidentally, it was necessary to pass by the waiting room where all of the other family members were gathered. Apparently, for some technical reason, the doctor and nurses found they had to make a brief stop at this point. Everyone was able to get a good look at Megan and Shannon. Needless to say, we were all quite pleased.

The twins arrived in the neonatal ward amidst a flurry of activity. Everyone was busy setting up appropriate monitors, respirators and other equipment. In addition, they were preparing the girls for ultrasonic and x-ray examinations. The transport team from Children's would be there in less than two hours, and there was quite a bit of information yet to be gathered.

I left Sandi and followed the girls to Neonatal. When I arrived, I noticed that some of the staff had paused for a second or two at the girls bed. Once I saw the twins, I realized why. After getting cleaned up, they had resumed the position that must have seemed most comfortable and safe to them. They had their arms around one and other. Not like they were dancing or hugging, but more like buddies.

That scene will remain vivid in my mind for as long as I live. Wendy took a Polaroid shot of the girls at about that same time. It was to become the most definitive of all the photos taken. To this day, people seeing it for the first time usually have very little to say. That picture tells the whole amazing story.

In the midst of all the activity, there were eight family members, anxiously waiting to see and touch Shannon and Megan. Phyllis, our case worker, was very helpful and understanding. She coordinated the visits by family members, and even bent the rules a little to provide everyone an opportunity. This included Helen, Tanja and Tom.

Those first visits to the girls were rather short, but very sweet and quite touching. It was all handled well.

While the rest of the family visited their new sisters, I performed some video taping. Not that we felt anything might go wrong, but we wanted to have lots of pictures and film of the twins early on, so that the explanations, which we were sure would one day be required, could be made with visual back-up.

Sandi was brought into the room on a gurney, straight from post-delivery surgery. She had talked them into letting her stop by on the way to recovery. She looked upon her new daughters through eyes that, although heavy with sedation, still beamed with love and joy.

I couldn't help but notice the rather large number of doctors and nurses passing by or stopping to deliver some small article or bit of information. I realized that many of them were there only to see the girls. Some, which I had never previously met, had actually been involved with Sandi and/or the twins in one way or another. A number of them did introduce themselves as they came or went, and I really was glad to meet them. I was still floating pretty high, and it would have taken a lot to dampen my spirits. I didn't care if everyone in the hospital made some sort of excuse to come see our daughters. I was happy for the safe delivery, and proud of my girls. Besides, everyone who came by was polite and courteous. They all seemed to comment on how beautiful and how perfect Shannon and Megan were.

The transport team arrived quickly. It must have been two hours later, but it sure didn't seem like it. All of the family's visiting was completed, and I was coming back down to earth. The first major objective, a successful delivery, had been achieved. The second, and more serious, was yet to come. I watched as the transport team prepared the girls for the ambulance ride across the Chicago suburbs. I wouldn't be going with them, but rather following in my car. The nurses informed the team from Children's, that Mom was to see the babies once more before they departed. We headed upstairs, to say good-bye to Sandi. Although the twins were all wired-up and tucked-in, the transport team was good enough to allow Sandi to hold and snuggle them before they began their journey.

At this time, the anesthesiologist who had been present in the delivery room, made a very touching and memorable comment. "I've been at many births," she said, "but it's been a very long time since I cried at one. It was so special, they are such little angels."

She was one of the many doctors and nurses who fell in love with twins immediately, treated them tremendously well, and did not want to see them leave. A number of the staff members at Lutheran General made the comment that we could always bring the babies back after the separation. They felt that they could take care of Megan and Shannon just as well as the staff at Children's from that time on. They were probably correct, but just then we had other things to occupy our minds.

Sandi bid a tearful good-bye to our new daughters. "I can't wait until I hold one of you in each arm," she said. With that, Shannon and Megan disappeared into the hospital elevator. I was able to relax at little, at that point. They were stable and appeared healthy. Hopefully, in the two or three days before the separation, they would grow even stronger, increasing the chances for successful surgery.

With the twins on their way, it was my turn to get moving. I said good-bye to Sandi, gathered up Helen, Laura and Tom, and headed for Chicago.

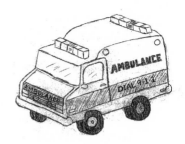

CHAPTER 9

The Next Event

I don't know what route the transport team took to get to Children's, but unless they had the siren turned on, it must have taken quite a while.

I had never been to this particular hospital before, but had received some pretty good directions on how to get there. We made the journey in just less than one hour. Most of the way there we talked about the twins, how good they looked, and how helpful everyone had been. It was amazing, however, to feel the change that came over us when Children's Memorial Hospital came into sight. What happened, I believe, was that we once more began to shift our thinking from the successful delivery, to the upcoming separation. Although I was sure I could handle everything okay myself, I really wished Sandi was there with us. I knew, beyond a shadow of a doubt, that she was wishing the same.

Getting the babies checked in was not too difficult. The hospital knew I was coming, and had most everything ready in the admissions area.

They have a security system there which requires all parents and visitors to be identified with passes. After receiving ours, and completing all the necessary admission paperwork, we headed up to the neonatal intensive care unit to meet the staff and see the twins.

Megan and Shannon were still being prepared for their stay, so we were shown around the unit by one of the nurses. We saw where the twins would be prior to and following surgery. I was concerned that after separation, they would be placed in two different locations within the unit. We really wanted to have them where we could visit them simultaneously. It was explained to us that proper space, with all the right equipment available, was somewhat limited, but they would do their best to get them together as soon as possible. I smiled to myself when I thought about it. All the trouble we were going through to successfully separate them, and I was trying to get them back together.

After our mini-tour, I was told that a Doctor Larry Moss would be meeting with me in a few minutes. He was, they explained, the Chief Fellow at Children's. He was in his final year, and would be performing the surgery along with Doctor Luck and Doctor Raffensperger.

While we were waiting to meet this doctor, more x-rays, ultrasonic examinations and blood tests were being processed on Shannon and Megan. Things were proceeding just about as we had expected they would.

We were ushered to a small, quiet room to wait for Doctor Moss. After ten minutes or so, he arrived. He appeared to me to be a bit nervous as he shook my hand

and introduced himself. Under the circumstances, I guess that was to be expected. What really wasn't expected, however, was what he had to say to me following the introductions.

"The girls have been stabilized and are alright," he said. "We want to operate right away. It appears they both have a bowel obstruction."

I don't think I even let him finish what he was saying, he had certainly taken me by surprise. "I thought it would be two or three days before you would operate," I said.

The doctor looked me straight in the eye and explained that If we waited, the twins would only get weaker, instead of stronger. That would surely diminish their chances.

I was still a little shook-up. For some reason, it had not dawned on me that they might need to proceed immediately. Operating now would, of course, mean that there was no way Sandi could make it to be with the girls and I for the surgery. It wouldn't matter how well anyone thought she might heal. There was just no way Lutheran General would let her leave within the twenty-four hour period following her own major surgery. It wasn't going to be fun telling her this.

For now, I wanted to know what exactly Doctor Moss meant by "right away", and asked.

"Just as soon as we can get it scheduled, most likely early tomorrow morning," he said. I also inquired as to when he might know the specific time. He told me to come back to the hospital 8:00 A.M. the next day.

He then talked with us a little more about the surgical procedure itself. We had some additional questions for him as well. Had anything changed from what we had originally believed? Did we know any more, now that the additional tests had been performed? He explained to us that they saw nothing significant enough to change the plans for Megan and Shannon. The hospital would be running more tests early in the morning, but basically, it looked as though the operation would consist of surgical division of the liver, and some additional work on the bowels. There were still some things they would not know until they got inside the two little bodies. For one thing, they had no idea how much bowel was there, and how it was shared. Secondly, they still didn't know how many bile ducts were present and where. They would have a much better idea the next day, after surgery had begun.

Doctor Moss was doing his best to be honest with me, and help me to understand just what the situation was. He was necessarily serious, however, and the implication of possible negative outcomes seemed only too evident.

He concluded our discussion with some general information about the operation and the medical team that would be involved. To be completely honest, I don't really remember much of what he did say at that time. My mind was sort of stuck on the image of my daughters going in for the surgery that would, one way or another, have an enormous effect on their futures. The day we had feared yet anticipated, dreaded but planned for, was at hand.

I walked out of that room torn between joy and sorrow. I was very happy that it was finally going to happen. Our little angels would, from now on, be beautiful but separate. The thought of all the pain and suffering yet to come, however, filled my heart with sorrow.

We walked back to the Neonatal Intensive Care Unit (NICU) to see the girls one more time. By now they had settled in and were resting peacefully. I kissed them both and headed to the nurses' station where they were to supply us with more information about the hospital and NICU. Mostly, it was to involve the issues of who could visit, when and how. They were, it turned out, quite particular about scrubbing-up and sterilization. We were told we would not be able to touch one of the babies and then the other, without scrubbing with hot water and soap in between. It would be all to easy to pass germs otherwise. It felt good to know they were taking every precaution. We thanked the nurses, said goodnight and headed out the door.

Before I had left Lutheran General, Sandi had told me not to come back later that evening, as I had planned. She wanted me to stay with the girls as long as possible, and then come see her in the morning; probably before visiting Shannon and Megan. She felt she would be too drowsy to be good company for me that night, and it would be quite late by the time I returned in any case.

As we walked toward the doors of Children's Memorial, I realized she had been correct. At the rate we were going, it would be after 10:30 by the time I could get back to her. I would go home and stay for the night.

There were relatively few people in the front lobby at this time, and we really weren't paying much attention to those who were present. We couldn't help but hear, however, part of a phone conversation which was taking place in the reception area. I don't remember the exact words, but it sounded something like this: "Yes, Fanning. They're here now. They arrived sometime this afternoon."

At the time, I figured it was just someone from Children's confirming the arrival of the twins with someone else from Lutheran General. It didn't seem all that inappropriate, even if it may have been happening a little late. I glanced at Helen, and figured that she had heard the same thing as I. Apparently she didn't feel it was unusual either. I decided it really didn't make much difference what it was about. The twins were safe and sound for now, and there hadn't been anything to suggest that any but the necessary few individuals knew that there were newborn, conjoined twins somewhere in Children's Memorial Hospital, awaiting separation.

I had already called Sandi from Chicago, to tell her of the change regarding the surgery. Even drugged and drowsy, her emotions came through. Similar to me, she was glad the time had come, yet worried over the possible outcome. As I had anticipated, she was quite upset that we would be apart for it all. There was just no way, however, she would have me anywhere but as close to our daughters as possible during the operation. I was glad that the drugs had made her so drowsy. I hoped they would help her get more sleep than I would that night.

When I returned home, there was a phone message from Children's. They wanted me to phone at about 7:00 A.M., to verify the time of the surgery. No problem, I thought, I might still be up by then anyway. Sleep will not likely come easy this night. As it turned out, the sheer exhaustion I was experiencing from such an emotionally active day, did help me sleep a little.

The next morning I awoke excited, anxious and physically rested. I really had a feeling that the day would have a positive ending. I knew that nothing had changed from the previous day. The chances for completely successful surgery had not increased. The girls still had bowel obstructions. We were still talking about a major surgical procedure to separate conjoined twins, perform major liver and bowel surgery (including possible intestinal reconstruction and/or re-routing), and put each of them back together as a complete, functioning child. When I thought about it too much, I began to wonder just why I felt so positive about success.

Laura arrived at 6:45 that morning. I had called her after listening to my phone messages the previous night. We had pre-arranged to leave from my house, stopping to pick up Helen on the way to Chicago.

The weather was a little cool, but not really all that unpleasant. It was a Friday, and I was glad we were getting away early. The traffic would be very heavy later that morning.

We arrived at the hospital between 7:30 and 7:45. Traffic had been pretty good, and we had no trouble finding a good spot in the hospital parking lot. The crossing light was red, and we were thus forced to wait at the street while traffic passed.

Looking across and up at the hospital, I couldn't help but think how much different it looked this morning. It appeared to be friendly enough. Yet at the same time, it sent the image of an imposing institution, somehow carrying the formula for life or death within it's very walls. I made an attempt to shake off the "image", and walked across the street to the hospital entrance.

With my thoughts focused more specifically on my daughters and the upcoming surgery, we headed through the front doors of Children's Memorial and presented ourselves at the reception desk.

I was glad to see that I was, apparently, being treated the same as any other parent. I told the gentleman at the desk that I was a parent, and showed my pass. He asked my name and I told him. He looked at a large file on the desk and said "which one?"

"Pardon me," I replied.

"Which one," he said again. "We have two here, Megan and Shannon. Which one are you here to see?"

"They're both my daughters," I replied.

"Oh, I see," he said. "I guess they're right next to each other anyway."

We walked on past the security guard, to the elevator that would carry us to the eighth floor and NICU.

Even at this early hour, the department was buzzing. There seemed to be an awful lot of hospital traffic. We found the door to the girls room, went in and began scrubbing-up. It started to become obvious, about then, that a good portion of the "traffic" was there because of the twins.

When we neared their bed, we ran into a crowd of doctors, technicians, nurses and interns. The shift nurse took us to the side and began explaining everything to us. They were still running some tests, while discussing the results of other tests already completed. It seemed as though the nurse was trying to keep us far enough away from the crowd so that we would not be able to hear the details of their conversation. I, on the other hand, was straining my ears to hear as much of what they were saying as possible.

As it turned out, it would have been better to shut out the crowd, and pay closer attention to what the nurse was trying to tell us. The doctors and technicians hadn't been saying anything I didn't already know anyway; and I felt a little silly asking the nurse to repeat what she had just said because I hadn't been listening. Eventually, though, I did get a full update from her.

They were going to take the twins downstairs to the operating room sometime between 9:00 and 9:30. There would be considerable preparation required, and it would take between two and two and one half hours. As far as the operation itself was concerned, Doctor Raffensperger would be talking to us in about thirty minutes. In the meantime, we could visit with the girls if we so desired. Of course we did desire to, and stayed there with them until it was time to talk to the doctor.

I believe Doctor Raffensperger not only wanted to explain what was going to take place in the operating room, but also wanted to ease my nervousness a bit. He presented the information to me in a way that not only showed the seriousness of the situation, but also told me he was confident of the ability of the operating room staff to complete the procedures successfully. He went over the general steps to be taken. The girls would first be separated, of course. This meant cutting through the abdominal walls, determining as best possible, just where organs, blood vessels and other items were located; and then cutting the liver more or less in two. Since the intestines may have also been joined, some cutting and re-routing might be necessary. Once all of this had taken place, one of the twins would be moved several feet to another operating table. All of the remaining work would be performed by two separate teams, one for each twin.

The remaining surgery would include correction of any bowel obstruction, reattachment of the bowel, possibly some bile duct work, and the closing of the abdominal wall. That was about it. Hopefully, there would be enough skin and tissue to cover such a large area.

He did say that if everything went well, the scars would heal quickly and not prove to be too ugly. "Of course, they will not have belly buttons, but they're only good for three things anyway. The first is catching lint. Then, little boys use them for holding flags in a parade, while girls store jewelry in them. And, of course, they're a good place for adults to keep the salt for their tequila.

"We can always make belly buttons for the girls in a couple of years, if you wish. We make real cute ones."

This little bit of humor he had added made us all smile. I believe that's what he intended to do, relax us a bit. We appreciated his effort, and I guess it did help some. The facts could not be denied, however. He knew and we knew, that this was very serious business; quite simply a matter of life and death.

Having provided us with the necessary details, he then

attempted to answer whatever questions we might have had. There weren't many. I asked him how long after surgery we could see the girls and he said "right away." I also wanted to know how long it might take to know if everything had been successful. He stated that usually the first 48 hours would be critical; but that it might be seven to ten days before we would know for sure.

Once Doctor Raffensperger had answered our questions, we were ready to go downstairs to see the area where the surgery would take place. The doctor had taken it upon himself to, more or less, be our guide.

He led us to a staff elevator which provided much quicker access to surgery via a less crowded route. When we reached the appropriate floor, he pointed out the surgical wing and the adjacent area. It was made clear to us that the choice of waiting areas was ours.

The large room we had just visited was also used as a waiting area for outpatient activity. It provided lots of room, comfortable furniture, but virtually no privacy. Upstairs, just adjacent to NICU, there was a smaller, more private waiting room, which might be used by other parents, but would never have more than a couple of families present. In addition, we had been offered the use of the "quiet" room where we had first met with the doctors. It was quite small, but offered privacy.

I talked it over briefly with Helen and Laura. It was an easy decision. We all wanted to be as close to the girls as possible. We would wait in the large room downstairs. Maintaining privacy, I felt, would be up to the three of us.

After the doctor finished showing us the way around

and explaining how we might best handle the wait, we headed back to the twins. We had brought both the video camera and the 35 mm. Since Sandi couldn't be there for another day or so, I was going to take pictures and do a little filming. So far, I had done nothing. One reason was that I had been too involved in other, more necessary things. Additionally, however, I felt quite uneasy about the concept. It seemed, somehow, to make the whole situation a little less serious and a little more theatrical. The truth was, though, not matter how it seemed, I knew I would regret having nothing to show Sandi regarding the twins' first two days at Children's and nothing to help document this part of our little angels' beautiful story. I retrieved my camera case, checked the batteries and headed into NICU.

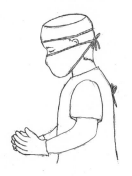

CHAPTER 10

The Surgery

The neonatal unit was still buzzing when I visited Megan and Shannon for the last time that morning. By then it was 9:00 A.M. and the girls were being prepared for surgery.

As promised, we took some still camera shots and a little 8mm footage. The twins were now sporting new toques (knit caps), a green one for Shannon and a pink one for Megan. Even with the medical apparatus that was now attached, they looked so healthy, peaceful and content. I wondered if I would ever again see them both that way. I wanted desperately to, not just believe, but really know that I would. After all, it was what we all had been hoping and praying for.

It was now just about time to begin the journey downstairs to surgery. There was, however, some additional

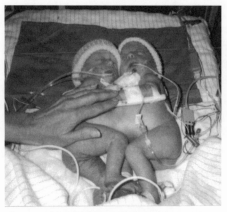

Shannon and Megan as they appeared after delivery, and prior to surgery. They were tiny, and obviously joined, but they looked beautiful and quite healthy.

information the medical staff needed to pass on to us.

First, we were introduced to the anesthesiologists who would be taking care of the girls. Then we were told who would be reporting the surgical progress to us and when.

We looked again at the area where the twins would be brought following surgery. Unlike Lutheran General's, their Neonatal unit was actually a series of small rooms. This setup seemed to allow for greater patient and family privacy.

Before we left, we saw where staff members had signed up to be on one or the other's team after surgery. It was really sort of touching. The nurses had prepared and hung posters welcoming each of the girls. Just looking at them, we got the feeling that Shannon and Megan would indeed be in competent, loving hands. They were happy little posters, made with care; the name of one twin and the appropriate nurses appearing on each. I knew that, in a day or two, when Sandi was able to come to there, she would be satisfied that our daughters were being properly cared for.

With all of the preliminaries seemingly settled, it was at

last time to head downstairs for the surgery.

The journey was a relatively quiet one, and I found time to continue the prayers I had begun earlier that morning. Since the first ultrasound had indicated a possibility of conjoined twins, I had offered the very same petition on a daily basis. Now that I had seen and touched my daughters, the intensity and passion of my plea could only increase. I knew God was listening. I knew he had heard me. The question was: in what way would my prayers, and those of so many friends and family members, be answered? To what degree would the surgery be successful? I expected we would have a good idea of the answer to this last question, before the sun had set that same day.

As we would have expected, the area outside surgery was fairly busy. There were a lot of medical people passing through the large double doors that led into the wing. I wasn't sure just how far they would let me go. It seemed that the area beyond those doors might be off limits to all but medical associates.

The gurney carrying the twins was stopped just outside the entrance, so that family members could say good-bye. Laura and Helen were still there with me. None of us really wanted to let the girls go any farther. I knew that what I did want at that time, more than anything else, was to take them in my arms, hold them close and just tell them that everything would be alright. Instead, I found myself touching and talking to them much like I would have, had they been Leanne and Laura. I was having a real problem holding back the tears, and even though they probably wouldn't know the difference, I didn't want to be crying all over them as they left. I would rather have them "feel" some strength and assurance from the person they would later know as Dad.

To ease the emotions welling up inside of me, I grabbed the recorder and began shooting. I really did want to get the girls on film right up to the point they were taken into the operating room. More than that, however, I just felt that keeping myself occupied in such a fashion would help prevent the tears from falling. There would be plenty of time to cry after the surgery had begun. I still had to call Sandi as soon as the girls went in, and I really needed to be in control. She would be relying on me to relate all the necessary information and to be here and ready if critical decisions needed to be made quickly. I wasn't going to let her, or my daughters down.

I finished filming, placed one hand on each of the twins and whispered a final prayer.

The time had come. The door to the operating room opened, revealing a small portion of the personnel and equipment to be used during the delicate surgery ahead.

I watched with mixed emotions, as our twin daughters, joined at the abdomen, disappeared into the unknown. The door closed quietly, almost solemnly, in front of me. Unable to go any farther, I walked back to Laura and Helen. We just stood there for a few seconds, not sure where we should go right then.

"If you guys want to sit down in the waiting room, go right ahead," I said. "I'm going to call Sandi and let her know they've started." With that, I walked down the hall to the nearest pay phone, drew a deep breath and dialed Lutheran General.

To say that Sandi had been anxiously waiting for my call, would have been a drastic understatement. The phone didn't even seem to ring before she answered. "Well," she said. "What's going on? How are they?" I explained all that had transpired since we last talked. "The girls were just fine when they took them into the operating room," I said. "They've just started the procedure, so we haven't received any update yet. I'll call you just as soon as I know anything. Try not to worry, they're going to be fine."

I made sure that everything I said came out sounding as positive as possible. She was relying on me to paint a true picture of what was happening. There was just no way I was going to sound apprehensive or unsure in the least.

"How are you doing?" I asked. "Are you going to be well enough to be with us in a day or so?" She said they had told her it would probably be Monday before she would be allowed to leave, but she was working on getting Doctor Pielet's approval for Sunday evening. She felt he knew us well enough to believe we would not do anything to jeopardize her health. I knew that he also realized she would not leave him alone until he released her. I figured there was a real good chance I could pick her up late Sunday.

Engaging in small talk, even with my own wife, was difficult at the time. For one thing, it was really hard to concentrate on any other subject for any length of time. I even found praying to be much more difficult than normal, so I had been keeping it short and simple. God knew what I was praying for, and he would understand.

There was, however one issue that Sandi and I had left hanging on several occasions. It was on the subject of the media, if and when we would talk to them, and how much we should tell them. A number of friends and relatives had commented that it would only be a matter of time until someone leaked the story.

We had been very lucky so far. An awful lot of people knew about the girls. How long could we expect them to maintain the secrecy? As one of our friends had cautioned, if they're going to find out, you should tell them yourselves, so at least the information is correct.

I decided to ease into the issue gradually with Sandi. "I have to call work and let them know what's going on," I said. "We've already had a couple of phone calls (on the beeper), a lot of people really want to know what's happening. I'm going to have to bring someone up to date. I think we might also have to consider talking to someone about the media. It's only a matter of time until somebody else does."

As I had expected, she didn't really want to talk about it right then. Her mind was on other things. Before our phone conversation ended, however, we had come to a decision. Since I was closer, physically, to the surgery and thus more likely to know first if the media or anyone else had found out about the girls, I would make the decision of when to release information. Before releasing it, I would call her and let her know. We also decided who we thought would be best to act for us in making the initial contact. We chose an associate of ours whom we knew would not have a problem talking to the press.

The whole issue of communicating with the media still didn't seem like a big deal. We figured they would probably check with the hospital and possibly send somebody over to get the story. Our phone conversation on the subject served largely as a diversion from more serious matters. I didn't feel we would need to talk much about it from then on.

I walked back to the waiting room to check on Laura and Helen. It was easy to see we were all still adjusting to the situation. They weren't quite ready to sit back, relax and wait, and I wasn't ready to stray more than a few feet from the doors to the operating room. I needed to be as close to my daughters as possible. I figured the walk to the pay phones was about the maximum I was willing to go right then.

That morning I had put on some loose-fitting, casual clothes and my most comfortable gym shoes. As it was turning out, I made the right decision. So far, I had spent the majority of my time standing or pacing. It certainly didn't look like that was going to change in the next few hours.

After we had been waiting for an hour or so, I was contacted by Erin Shields, the hospital's media services representative. She had received a phone call from a local station, asking for a statement about the twins. Apparently, someone had talked. She wanted to know what, if anything, we wanted to release. I told her I would talk to Sandi and get back to her. It still didn't seem to be a big deal, they weren't exactly beating the doors down to interview us. I called Sandi and explained the situation to her. The decision was an easy one. It was time to have someone talk to the media, giving them as little information as possible, while making sure the facts were correct. As it turned out, that was to be much easier said than done.

I decided to call work. I had promised to give our engineering staff assistant an early update. I also wanted to talk to one of the engineers, and have him pass on some limited information to a local TV station. Before I had a chance to complete my call, however, the news had hit the air. At least one radio station had released it as a breaking news story. I spoke to several of our friends on the phone, and found that some of them had heard the story on the radio. Apparently, however, some of the facts were incorrect.

That did it. I called our contact, went over all the key information, and asked him to release just what we had discussed to a particular local TV station. "Are you sure you want me to do this?" he asked, well aware of the fact that we were trying to maintain as much privacy as possible. I told him that Sandi and I had just discussed it, and the time was right. He wasted little time in making the first contact.

From then on, things got rather crazy. There was considerably more interest than we had anticipated. Erin Shields called me on the beeper. They had now received numerous phone calls from radio stations, newspapers and television stations. She thought we should release a brief statement, so that everyone would get the same information at the same time. As strange as it may seem, I hadn't really thought about that. I was a little embarrassed, to now realize that this was probably why media services contacted me in the first place. They were better able and at least as willing to handle all media issues while we were there at the hospital.

I explained to Erin what I had already released, and to whom. She didn't think it would pose any problem. She believed however, that we needed to determine very quickly just how much we were willing to release. She cautioned me that some of the media people would pursue every possibility to get additional material. This would be especially true if they truly considered this a lead story. We decided to release of the following: Information on the twins (names, sex, date of births, place of births), and information on the parents (names, city in which they live). We were also willing to admit the twins were presently undergoing separation surgery.

This did not seem like an awful lot of data, but I really thought the media would accept it for now. They would surely realize, I rationalized, that there would be more information provided later on. This way, I felt, some of our privacy, and certainly most of other family members' privacy, would remain protected. It didn't take long to discover I had been quite wrong.

I should have been glad that everything with the media was happening so quickly. It should have helped take our minds off of the twins and the surgery; but it didn't. Oh I guess that each phone call I placed or received did, temporarily, interrupt my thoughts about what might be happening the other side of those double doors. The thoughts always returned quickly, however, not allowing any time for relaxing.

It's difficult to explain just how I was feeling. On the outside, I was alert and sharp; waiting, listening watching and pacing. On the inside, however, I was churning with a variety of emotions. I had never experienced anything like this in my life. I continued to pray for my daughters off and on. I hoped God was listening and understanding. My offerings, I knew, must have seemed disjointed and somewhat erratic, even to the almighty one. Some of the time I just seemed to be repeating "Dear God" and "please" over and over. There was little doubt that my plan to remain calm and strong through it all, might be coming undone.

Knowing what I went through, I can only imagine how difficult it must have been for Sandi. Thankfully, some friends of ours, Terry and John, were with her at Lutheran General. Since we hadn't planned on the surgery taking place so soon, we hadn't arranged for this in advance. They had just decided on their own, as soon as they knew she would be alone.

Sandi called my beeper again. It didn't seem like it had been that long since we last spoke. To her, however, each minute must have seemed like hours. She needed reassurance that everything was still alright. I had not heard any more from the operating room, and told her so. She seemed quite concerned, so I explained to her that it probably would be difficult and unwise for anyone to be coming and going during such a delicate operation. I suspected they would wait until an appropriate time, when the individual leaving the room would not be missed and would not disturb any other medical personnel still involved in the surgery. She agreed with me to some degree, while I began to wonder why I had not been updated. Based on what I had been told, I expected to be updated no later than three hours after the start of surgery. The twins had been in there for at least two hours, and we had heard nothing yet. I told her I was sure everything must be okay, and that I probably should wait a while longer before looking for someone to give us an update.

"By the way," Sandi said, "we have apparently been all over the radio and television. From what I've heard, they don't have all the information correct. What did you tell them anyway? Tanja says that they have called the house, and even sent someone with a camera over."

I explained to her just what we had released. Obviously, I had misjudged the newsworthiness of our story, as well as the resourcefulness of the media. Somehow they had found where we lived. I decided I had better call Tanja and provide her with instructions on how to handle the phone calls.

Tanja, it turned out, had been very busy. Before filling me in, however, she wanted to know if we had any news on the girls. I explained the situation to her, and then listened as she related information on the numerous phone calls she had received.

There had been calls from several of the TV stations and two newspapers. In addition, there had been some unidentified callers. Tanja also explained that someone from one of the TV stations had been there with a camera. At the time, Paul was the only one home. When he saw who was at the door, he refused to answer it. Apparently, they shot some footage anyway, and my son's backside ended up as part of a "live, breaking story." Later on, Sandi and I were to both get a real chuckle out of that.

I asked Tanja if she had heard from anyone else. She said that my daughter Leanne had called. She wanted to check on the twins, but also wanted to know if we had given her name and number to the media.

I told Tanja that we absolutely had not, which was what she had figured anyhow. Someone had, however, found out that Leanne Pankuch was my daughter, and called her with questions about her twin sisters. I found that to be rather amazing at the time, and even a little scary. Boy! had I ever underestimated their resourcefulness.

I told Tanja to hang in there, and let the answering machine handle the calls. I would take care of replies when I got home. With that, I headed back to the waiting area to see if the doctor might be looking for me. I really wanted to hear some good news.

When I got back to the waiting room, there appeared to be some commotion going on. Helen and Laura pointed out what everyone seemed to be so interested in. There were two different TV news trucks parked alongside the hospital. The people in the room were discussing just why they might be there. We made no comment, and walked back out into the hall. We all had already guessed they were most likely here for the twins' story.

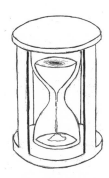

CHAPTER 11

The Wait

I don't recall just when I realized I had memorized the color combination and the pattern for the entire surgical entry hall, but when it struck me, I knew it was time to find some activity other than pacing to pass my time.

Once we had noticed the television trucks, I felt I really didn't want to stay in the waiting room with the other parents. I guess I thought they might figure out who I was. As it turned out, however, I began to notice that most of the families weren't staying long anyway. They seemed to be coming and going every hour or so. By 11:00, there were only two families remaining who had been there since we arrived. Most, apparently, had been there for outpatient surgery. Once I realized that fact, I felt a little safer, and re-entered the waiting room with Laura and Helen.

None of us had eaten breakfast yet that morning, and we were already starting to feel the effects. We really needed some food to help sustain us during the long wait. I told the others to go ahead and get something, I would wait there in case we got some early news.

It turned out to be necessary for them to return to our van for some item we had inadvertently left there. They promised, however, to avoid the media if at all possible. The visitors passes they were wearing had the patients' names written on them, so it was necessary to cover them as soon as they passed through the hospital doors.

Their little excursion went smoothly. They returned in a few minutes with some food for all of us. No one had questioned or otherwise bothered them. We all felt good about that. I don't believe any of us was yet ready to discuss the twins.

We weren't supposed to bring food into the waiting room, but I wasn't about to leave. So, we did something I don't normally do a lot of. We broke a rule.

As we ate, Helen explained that the reporters had been questioning virtually all the medical personnel leaving the hospital. She had caught a portion of one conversation in passing. Apparently, they were asking some nurse about the girls. She replied that she knew the twins were in the hospital and in surgery, but nothing else.

We spent a little time talking about the media, what they knew, when and how. During this conversation, something dawned on me. Just maybe that phone conversation we had heard a portion of the night before, had not been with Lutheran General at all. As a matter of fact, it made sense that it most likely had indeed been with someone else.

Well, it didn't matter now. Surgery was well underway,

and no matter how hard any media personnel might try, they would not be able to get near the operating room. As a matter of fact, from what we had seen, they would be lucky to get in the hospital at all.

We figured that, since the media was so interested, and one of the television news trucks had been there for hours, maybe we should make an attempt to see what they had to say on television. But when we thought again, it became apparent that It might just upset us instead. We didn't need that. Television could wait.

I talked to Sandi again. "Still no news," I explained. "I'm going to try and find someone from surgery if I don't soon hear something."

The time continued to pass. Some of it went quickly, but most of it dragged by. I kept busy with numerous phone calls. Several additional conversations took place with Sandi, but most of the calls, in one way or another, involved the media. They had really picked up the ball. Several radio and television stations now had us as a breaking story. Although they had been given all the correct information, which we had at that time wanted to release, it seemed as though many of them had still gotten some facts incorrect. The name Sharon seemed to have become quite popular, for instance. One report had given this name to the twins' mother, while another report gave the same name to one of the twins. I was actually feeling good about the fact that I had not yet seen or heard any news reports myself.

It was now after 12:00, and we had settled on believing that the medical staff was just too busy and concerned with the more important things to send someone from the operating room to see us. We were sitting quietly in front of the television, just sort of staring at it without really paying any attention.

The inevitable then happened. The noon news report had come on, as we sat there. There didn't seem to be a lot of sense in getting up and running out just to miss it. That probably would have drawn some unwanted attention from the other parents anyway, so we watched. The coverage they gave us was brief, but they promised a full story later that afternoon. This broadcast, at least, seemed to have the facts correct.

The other parents present showed a lot of interest when they discovered that the surgery was taking place at Children's. The three of us just looked at one and other and smiled weakly. At that point there wasn't a lot else we felt we could or wanted to do.

While we were still waiting for initial word, I decided to make a few more phone calls. I wanted to talk to key family members, to let them know not to expect any calls from us until after the surgery had been completed later that day. The way I figured it, there was no need to have all those other people worry unnecessarily.

The noon hour had now come and gone. The television trucks remained outside the building, and only one other family was still there from the initial morning group. I supposed that they must also have been waiting out some complicated surgical procedure. From what I could tell, their group must have contained more family representation than ours.

Shortly after 1:00, I made contact with the desk in the surgical wing. They promised to check things out and have someone get back to me.

The next time I got on the phone with Sandi, she was terribly concerned. Doctor Pielet had called her to see how things were going with the twins. When he realized that we hadn't yet heard anything, he had offered to call over and see what he could do. She had told him to go ahead. I didn't mind. I just wanted to know. It didn't really matter much who was responsible for getting an update to us. I was sure the medical people were busy doing what was best for our daughter. In the meantime, however, they had some very worried parents getting more so all the time.

I, myself, had seen quite enough of the waiting area, and was even fast losing the ability to concentrate long enough to offer a prayer. Amazingly enough, up until then, I had maintained the ability to remain rather calm and collected on the outside, while dealing with all of the "what ifs" on the inside. I did need something, however, to refuel me physically and mentally. I had begun to let my emotions come to the surface. Sandi noticed it during that phone call. It was all too apparent that we really needed a positive update soon.

The next time the door to the waiting area opened, I just knew it was our update. I recognized the individual as one of the doctors from surgery. He immediately apologized and explained that the surgery had been a little late in starting. They had, as a matter of fact, performed a dry run prior to beginning. The actual surgery hadn't started until around 12:00, following the two and one half hours of preparation.

He went on to tell us that they were just beginning to separate the liver. Everything was going as planned, and they would let us know when the actual separation was complete.

Needless to say, we were greatly relieved. The surgery had not been going on for almost five hours, but rather closer to two. Apparently, the two and one half hours of preparation took place after the entered the operating room. There certainly had been some miscommunication. Regardless of what the staffing may have been trying to tell us, we all ended up understanding that this preparation took place before they entered the operating room. As a matter of fact, when we visited NICU between 7:00 and 9:30, we were told the girls were being prepared for surgery.

In any case, that didn't matter any longer. We all understood the situation as it then stood. There would be no more misunderstanding.

I phoned Sandi right away to explain what was going on. She, also, was relieved, but seemed somewhat disappointed. We had been hoping that the surgery would be just about over by that time. She mentioned that Doctor Pielet had reached someone in surgery. They, of course, were reluctant to release any information over the phone. After verifying his identity, they gave him a status update on the surgery. They also reassured him that someone would, get to me with an update. I told her to thank the doctor, but I certainly hoped that they had been preparing to update us even as he called.

Knowing that the surgery was going according to plan, and needing a change of atmosphere, Laura and I decided to slip out to the cafeteria for a quick bite.

Our lunch was short and uneventful. Neither of us had been all that hungry. On the way back from the cafeteria, however, it sure seemed as though a lot people were giving us long looks. I tried to determine whether they had figured out that we were the family of the conjoined twins, or they just wondered what such a nice young girl was doing with an older guy like me.

It suddenly struck me that this was another reason why this whole event was so very special. Here I was in the middle of the greatest emotional drama I had known, the very lives of my two infant daughters hanging in the balance, and some of my greatest and strongest support was coming from my two adult daughters.

I thought about the fact that some people go to their graves terribly saddened because their grown children had never told them that they loved them. I was much luckier than most. Leanne and Laura had already shown me all I ever needed to see. They would never have to say anything else.

We returned to Helen in the waiting area and continued the vigil.

My sister, always outgoing and helpful, had made friends with a young woman and her daughter. The little girl had been a patient there for many months, and seemed to enjoy the attention.

As Helen introduced them to us, I couldn't help but realize just how many such stories this hospital must go through each year. It had been, no doubt, a Godsend for many children and their families.

It wasn't just Children's Memorial. There must have been thousands of hospitals and clinics all around the world dedicated to providing happy, healthier, more bearable lives for children of every description. It was saddening to realize that there were so many children who needed help, but at the same time, heartening to know that so many people were willing to give that help. I thanked God once more for all the health and happiness my grown children had known, and asked him to allow Shannon and Megan the same opportunity.

Feeling a little more blessed and hopeful, I called my wife again. By this time, the families coming and going had virtually stopped. There were, basically, just the two families in the waiting room. The other family seemed serious enough about their wait, and I was not going to impose on them.

Three o'clock came and went. Tom came from work to finish the wait with us. That helped, as we had all been getting a little numb. Having a new face to look at, and someone else to discuss the situation with gave us a little new life. It had been a long day, and we had gotten only too use to waiting. The television news trucks were still outside. I thought maybe it was time we had a look at what they were saying about us. I knew one of the trucks was from a station which had been provided with our initial statement. It looked like it might be a good idea to turn the television over to that channel at 4:00.

The television had, for a good portion of the morning,

been set on another station. I had not really been watching it, and didn't know if anyone else had. Just prior to the hour, I asked the others in the room if they minded my changing the station. They were very nice about it, but said that they had been waiting for a special broadcast about something going on here at Children's. I glanced at the rest of my family, and replied, "okay, we'll watch that."

We were the headline story alright, a breaking news event. The first portion of the broadcast was pretty standard and about what we had expected. They announced that conjoined twins had been born yesterday afternoon, in Park Ridge, and were being separated today at Children's Memorial. Then, they gave the names of the twins and the parents. While it seemed a bit odd to hear our names on the news, it was really no big deal; nothing to get upset or excited about. That which followed, however, fell into a very different category.

Sandi had told me earlier, that the doctor who had given the symposium on conjoined twins had been on the radio. He apparently made some comment about knowing the twins were joined at the liver, but not being personally involved in the case. We had pretty much figured that most of the television and radio stations would be attempting to find their own "experts" on conjoined twins, so as to interview them on the air.

This station had found theirs. He was from North-western University and we had never heard of him. I don't say that to discredit the gentleman, but rather in order to help point out the fact that he was in no way involved in our case. The interview with this "expert" was short but far from sweet. He was first asked some general questions about conjoined twins; to which he gave the standard answers. Then, he was asked a more specific question regarding our girls. It went something like this: "Based on your knowledge of the Fanning case, what would you say these babies chances are?" He began his reply with a comment that our girls were in double danger; first of all because of the major surgery required (liver separation and bowel reconstruction). Secondly, due to the fact that they were delivered so many weeks prematurely. As a direct reply to the reporters question, he stated: "I believe their chances of survival are very poor."

This was more than outrageous. It was totally unbelievable, in my mind, that any doctor would be so irresponsible. I was not able to hold myself back. "You _____," I said rather quietly, using a slang term for a certain part of the human anatomy. "Just what do you know about the twins? What do you know about all the care and preparation that went into making sure they were healthy and strong when they were born?" By this time, tears had formed in my eyes. With all we had been going through, why did this have to happen? Why did he have to say that? I hoped that Sandi had not been watching the same program.

It took only a few seconds for my daughter to realize that this one thoughtless statement had managed to do what, up until then, had not seemed possible. It had broken my resolve to completely control my outward emotions in front of others. As my daughter comforted me, I shook my head and wept.

It's hard to explain just why this was demoralizing. I can just say that this doctor had caught us unprepared. We had known all along, that, without everything going just right, the twins would indeed be facing an uphill battle. So far, however, no medical person had ever stated that the chances of them surviving this surgery could be so poor. Everyone had either, just assumed success would occur, or had kept their opinions to themselves. Here was a supposedly knowledgeable doctor making an extremely negative statement without even having all of the facts. When you put this together with the fact that we had been waiting, almost desperately, to receive some word on the success of the surgery, perhaps you can understand the effect this report had on us. No matter how positive we had been, this gave some credence to any lingering thoughts we may have had about possible negative outcomes.

My sister had, obviously, also been upset. She was making comments about a professional doctor addressing an issue of which he knew nothing, while also, attempting to comfort me.

The other family in the waiting took only a few more seconds to realize what was going on. Helen spoke with them briefly and explained who we were. As it turned out, they had been going through some very difficult times as well. Their situation involved a young girl who had gone through one serious problem after another.

That day, her parents, grandparents, aunt and uncle were all there to help see her through yet another one. Once they knew who we were and realized our situation, they quietly offered their support and prayers.

One of the ladies, I believed to be the grandmother, offered me a special gift for Sandi. It was only a plastic, rosary that glowed in the dark, but she had prayed with it regularly for her granddaughter. She wanted us to have it now. It was a symbol of the faith and love that had helped hold their family together during those hard times. I took it from her gladly and promised to pass it on to my wife as soon as we saw one and other.

The idea of receiving such love and support from people we had only just met, was almost mind-boggling. I had no doubts about their sincerity. These were genuinely good people. Quite often, following the twins' surgery, I thought about that family. I later regretted not having remembered and saved their names. At the time, however, that did not seem really important. They were there with us only briefly, but offered a special kind of support that can only be provided by someone who has been there. Attempting to repay their generosity, I have prayed for them, and prayed for the beautiful little girl they had all come to Children's to support.

I knew I had to call Sandi again, before she heard about this newscast from someone else. First, however, it was necessary for me to make sure I had external control of my emotions. I accomplished this rather quickly and got on the phone to Lutheran General.

I broke it to Sandi as gently as I could. She was furious. She wanted to know who this guy was and what gave him the right to make such a statement. We talked it over for a while and decided the best we could do was to help the doctors at Children's and the twins show everybody how wrong this guy had been. We ended our conversation there, as I really felt like we would soon be receiving an update. I didn't want to be hard to find when that happened.

I realized that, no matter how quickly our update came, the events that had just transpired would make the remainder of the wait, the most emotionally difficult time we had thus far endured.

Before I returned to the waiting room, I got in touch with Erin Shields. I explained what we had seen on the television. She was quite upset and stated that she would call the TV station and Northwestern both immediately. That, at least, eased my mind a bit.

It wasn't long after I returned to the room that our update came. As I listened to hear what the doctor had to say, I could feel my heart pounding. "Oh please God, let it be good news" I whispered.

They had completed separation of the liver. Although it had taken longer than expected, everything had gone about as planned. The girls were now on separate operating tables, having individual surgery performed. It looked like they would finish up just after 5:00.

I looked into the doctor's face to see if I could detect any signs of emotion that might give some additional idea of how he thought things were going. There wasn't much there; if anything, maybe just of bit of relief. Apparently he, like us, would have to wait until sometime after the completion of the procedure.

I immediately got back on the phone and updated Sandi. We were both happy and relieved at what had transpired thus far. We knew at the time, however, that it wasn't over yet. They were still in surgery, and still subject to most of the same hazards. Though the doctors had been able to tell us that the separation was complete, they had not been able to say anymore about what they found once they got inside, let alone how it was handled. We would just have to be patient and wait until after 5:00 to hear the rest.

By the time I got off of the phone, it was nearly 5:00. We were all quite apprehensive, although actually feeling fairly positive. The doctor had made everything he described sound more or less routine, but that was his job. We were thinking that, if things had indeed gone as planned, then there would be some pretty happy and satisfied medical people around after five. We would be anxiously looking for those happy faces.

It wasn't long before one of the doctors returned. The surgery had basically been completed. Shannon would be coming out of the operating room in a few minutes. Megan was still being worked on and would follow several minutes later. Everything had gone well, and one of the surgeons would be up to talk with us in a little while.

The next few minutes went by very quickly. We asked a number of question and received somewhat general answers. It seemed as though both girls were alright, but we hadn't yet received any details.

As promised, Shannon came out first. She seemed to be almost covered with bandages, wires and tubes. Since she was on a gurney, and manual respiration was being applied, we could not get a close-up look at her. The medical team was not about to stop. They told me I could hop in the elevator with them if I wanted to, however.

They wanted to get the girls back to NICU and properly attached to all of the equipment as quickly as possible. That was alright with us. Megan followed her sister upstairs. She looked about the same as Shannon, except a little more swollen. Looking at both our daughters, I could only imagine what they had just been through. At least, I thought, they're both alive. At the same time, however, I remembered Doctor Raffensperger's words, "no one dies in the operating room." Surely, since the doctors had spent so much time on each of the girls, they were planning on both of them surviving the long term. It would be difficult indeed, to wait until I had heard all that the surgeons had to say.

The wait, was not all that long. Doctor Raffensperger seemed rather relieved. He explained several important things to us. First of all, he said that everything had gone well. Megan, however, had proven to be a bit of a problem as far as sedation was concerned. Since the girls were joined, they shared some circulation. This was in spite of the fact that each had her own circulatory system. It seemed whatever was administered to one, would, at least partially, end up in the other. That was a real problem. Some of the sedative meant for Shannon, was ending up in Megan's system. It turned out to be a delicate procedure to get both twins properly sedated.

They had found bowel obstructions in both girls. These were removed, and some additional surgery and reconstruction was required.

Another difficulty was presented by the positioning of

the babies. Because they were joined, and could not be laid flat on their backs, a good portion of the operation had to actually take place at a 90 degree angle. This took quite a bit of getting used to, and added some more time to the procedure.

The final concern, involved the biliary tracts. This is the system by which the bile, used in processing food, moves from the gallbladder through the intestines, the stomach, the large intestine, then out through the rectum. Although some bile excretion had been present, the doctors had been unable to positively identify the presence of a complete biliary tract in either baby. In Shannon, they had found a bile duct. With Megan, however, they had not been able to verify the presence of one. He felt however that chances of one being there were quite good.

I couldn't wait for anymore explanations. "When will we know for sure that everything is okay?" I asked. He explained that the next twenty-four to forty-eight hours would be critical. After that, we would be looking at another seven to ten days before we could be sure. There was still a possibility that, if all went well, we could take them home in four to five weeks.

The doctor had seemed genuinely positive about the whole procedure, so I didn't ask him to comment anymore about possible problems with Megan and her biliary tract. I knew, only too well, what might happen if that concern ended up in with a negative outcome.

We would continue to wait and pray. For now, our little angels were both alive; alive and separate. I called Sandi immediately with the news.

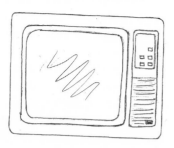

CHAPTER 12

Media Blitz

Erin shields had gotten in touch with me again prior to the completion of surgery. The media knew the twins were due out of the operating room around 5:00. They wanted to have a press conference. Erin realized that if we agreed, it would only be if everything had gone okay. Sandi and I had felt from the very beginning that this was going to be a happy story. We would have no problem sharing it with everyone else.

I spoke with Erin again after surgery. The plan was to have the conference here at the hospital, with one of the attending physicians and the father fielding questions. They would require about fifteen minutes from each of us. This would all take place at between 6:00 and 6:30. We didn't have all that much time.

Not long after Shannon had come out of surgery, Doctor Luck came up to us. I thanked her for what she had done and she acknowledged. There was something else on her mind, though. She seemed a bit upset. Apparently, they were making her do the press conference. She stated that she didn't think it was a good idea. I politely disagreed. She stated that she would go ahead and talk to the media, but didn't feel that I needed to at that time.

It was plain to see we weren't going to agree. She and the rest of the doctors had done a marvelous job. We were tremendously thankful for that. I knew they didn't like dealing with the media, but I didn't see any reason why I shouldn't.

I explained to her that I would not be answering any medical questions, only personal and/or family ones. She asked why I wanted to do this. I explained to her that the media already had some information and had been digging for more. It made sense to me to provide them what they needed, within reason, in a forum where we had some control. With that our conversation ended. I didn't know what to expect at the upcoming press conference, but I still respected and admired Doctor Luck and her associates. It appeared as though we owed them much.

While the twins were getting settled back in NICU, we spoke with some of the nurses. They were really happy to see that things appeared to have gone well. In addition, they knew about the press conference. Most of them had seen or heard something prior to coming in to work. They were calling the girls little celebrities and asking us if we were ready to go on television.

That was a good question. We hadn't really thought much about it. I certainly realized that I needed to have some idea of what to say, but I guess I just figured the right words would come. After what we had seen of the media that day, and what we remembered about some of the questions they had asked other families in such situations, we decided maybe we should take a few minutes to prepare.

Erin got in touch with me again. The press conference would be starting in just a few minutes. The plans had been changed just a little. Doctor Luck would go on first to answer questions for about 15 minutes. When finished, she would leave and I would take the podium. I would, most probably, spend about the same amount of time answering questions. That sounded fine to me.

They thought it would be a good idea for us to have some privacy prior to seeing the media. That way, we could prepare, if necessary, and they would know right where to find us when the time had come. We were, therefore, taken to one of the "quiet", family rooms to ponder the upcoming interview.

I should have been real nervous, but I wasn't. It was difficult to figure out just why. I certainly was not in any way used to being in front of reporters; this, obviously, would be my first time. The only reason I could imagine, was that, because we had just been over such an emotional roller coaster, I was spent. When I thought about it a little longer, I realized that the only emotions I was feeling right then were positive; relief, happiness, hope and love. The day had been so draining, there was just no room left for those negative ones. Heck, they were probably recuperating themselves.

This conference wouldn't be bad at all. I would go in

there happy and not at all nervous.

Laura and Helen felt that, while putting on a happy face might be considered preparation, it might also be worthwhile to think about what questions the media might ask. They were correct.

The most negative issue I could think of them bringing up was the age difference between Sandi and I. But, then again, they had never before seen either of us. They would have no idea I was that much older. That one would be no problem.

I was really feeling pretty good right then. Having been known to possess a fairly sharp wit and a good sense of humor, I did come up with a couple of "amusing" answers to questions we thought sure they might ask. Although I decided not to use them, I will say that knowing they were there, should the situation demand, made me feel even better.

The minutes continued to pass rather quickly. We were soon ushered downstairs to a small auditorium for the conference. Doctor Luck was still being interviewed when we entered, and I was able to listen to her final replies. It seemed as though she had done an admirable job. Now it was my turn.

Had anyone ever told me that I would one day stand in front of numerous television cameras and microphones, while experiencing absolutely no nervousness or fear, I would have told them they were crazy. Yet, early on the evening on March 25th, 1994, that's exactly what happened.

It was amazing. I could not believe how relaxed I really was. I wasn't emotionless, I smiled and possibly even blushed a little at a couple of comments. I was just plain cool and calm. If I could bottle whatever it was that affected me that way I would be a millionaire. It was great. Nothing they were going to say could at all phase me. I was in control.

"Have you seen your daughters since the surgery," they asked. "Yes," I replied. "What do you think of them now?"

"They're gorgeous. They were gorgeous when they were born, and they're gorgeous now, even though they're a little puffed-up and poked full of holes."

Those questions more or less set the stage. If they had wanted to hear something more dramatic, something about them looking like monsters before, but being beautiful after, they had the wrong father. I had meant just what I had said.

They did go on to ask a number of other questions, including one about our ages. I made some discretionary initial reply. Near the end of the interview, however, I did supply them with more or less exact information. I was afraid they might, otherwise, come up with some even more ridiculous disparity.

One question, which I should have anticipated, but didn't, was that regarding insurance. Were we insured they wanted to know. The answer was, of course, yes; but I really didn't know exactly what would and wouldn't be covered. It may have sounded illusive on my part, but I told the truth. I just didn't yet know.

When they had finished with me, they asked my daughter Laura for a comment. She happily obliged with a positive reply.

That was it. After the cameras shut down, there was a

period of informal conversation. A lot of congratulations were extended, and some introductions made. A few of the names I recognized from television; others I didn't. Some of the reporters asked to do follow-ups, or asked for some kind of exclusive.

I knew how Sandi felt about exclusives, and I felt the same. This was a happy story. We wanted to share it with everyone. All of the information we could provide would be shared. If there were some other kind of exclusive, we would be willing to talk about it later.

The conference had lasted quite a bit longer than fifteen minutes, by the time the informal portion had been concluded. I was getting quite tired, and still had a lot to do. With the media temporarily out of the way, I could get back to the twins.

When I got to the room and saw them again, they were doing fine. All of the support and monitoring equipment had been hooked up, and the nurses were right there with them.

As I looked at them, and softly touched their swollen bodies, I was brought back to reality. The apparent success of the surgery must have left me in some sort of state of euphoria. I felt extremely guilty about having left them so soon after the surgery, and about showing all my happiness to the press. I was still happy to see them, but that happiness was now mixed with extreme concern. Had I forgotten they were in critical condition and still far from being out of danger? I kissed them each gently, and asked them to forgive me.

I called Sandi and updated her on what had taken place at the press conference. John and Terry were still there with her, and would stay until I arrived. Since it was almost 8:00, I figured I wouldn't get there until about 9:00.

Laura, Tom and Helen headed for home, prepared to answer the many questions they would be receiving. I said good-bye to the twins, whispered a little prayer, and headed for the van.

I was anxious to get to Lutheran General to be with my wife. It had been a very long, very emotional day. I knew the twins were not out of danger, but at least we had cleared one enormously large hurdle.

The comment the doctor had made about not being able to find Megan's bile duct starting eating at me again, as I pulled out of Children's parking lot. Why couldn't it have been more simple. It would have been a lot nicer to have heard the doctor say "the girls are fine. Everything went perfectly. They both should live normal, full and happy lives, end of story." I reckoned, however, that those kind of endings really never take place, except maybe in the movies.

Hollywood takes an actual ending, happy or otherwise, that may have taken months to unfold, and compresses it into a happy ending taking less than one day. I guessed that, in our case, the waiting and praying would continue a while longer.

I was just turning onto the expressway, when the radio caught my ear. The announcer was saying "and in our lead story." Then, I heard a strangely familiar voice. It was my own. They were playing some of my statements back over the air. I listened to the reporter's comments and then to my reply. Hey! I thought. That's not exactly what they asked me. The answer they were playing had been meant for a different question. They only played a few seconds of the interview, but it was the beginning of what I can only describe as a somewhat disturbing pattern. By playing back my answers and attaching different questions, they could manipulate what I had said, or so it seemed. Some of the time their idea was to try and increase the drama, make it sound as though we needed money, or that we had already received significant monetary support. At other times, they really didn't manage to change the context all that much.

From listening to and watching these interviews, I was to learn an important lesson. From then on, each time I answered, I would do my best to word it so as not to be usable in any other context. It wouldn't be easy, and was not always possible, but I would try.

I managed to make fairly good time driving to Lutheran General. I was able to keep my mind mostly on the road, although there were al lot of other thoughts popping in and out of my head. I thought about Sandi quite a bit. I realized that she, most likely received a good number of phone calls herself today. In fact, since a lot of interested people did not know how to reach me, and she was confined to her hospital room, it was reasonable to assume she had received quite a few more than I had. My assumption turned out to be correct. Most of the calls she had received were from friends or relatives, looking for some additional information on the girls, or wanting to know how she was doing.

It seemed we had been all over the news. Most of the television stations had shown the girls and I briefly, and then stated that there would be a full story at 9 or 10:00.

There was one negative note regarding phone calls. Sandi's grandmother was one of the individuals from whom we had intentionally withheld the whole story. She was getting up there in years, and was not in the best of health. Sandi had told her we were expecting twins. She had not, however, told her that they were joined. She had discovered that by watching the news. To make matters worse, it had been the station with the "expert" from Northwestern. When she had heard his gloomy prediction, she had immediately phoned Sandi's parents. As it turned out, they had to call an uncle, who lives here in Illinois, to go over and take care of her. She was so upset, he had to stay with her all night.

I brought Sandi up to date as best I could regarding the twins and surgery. I tried to think of as many details as possible, so that she would have a true picture of everything. I avoided the issue of the media as much as possible. It was true that they had been a big part of that day, but that wasn't what it was all about. This was about our daughters, what they had been through, how they were doing now and what the current prognosis was. As we talked, I began to feel somewhat strange about being so far from the girls. Since their conception, one of us had always been within a few feet of both. Now we were miles away.

Sandi asked me again how the girls really looked, and I said "fine." I was glad that I had left the movie camera in the van. I didn't think it would be a good idea for Sandi to see what they looked like directly following surgery. It wouldn't really be fair. They needed to have a couple of days to recuperate. "You'll see them yourself in a day or so," I said. "You'll see that they are just fine." I collapsed in the chair next to the bed, too worn out to do much else. Sandi wanted to run the tape of the delivery, so that Terry could see it. I watched it also. Most of it I had already seen first hand, but it made me happy and proud to see it again.

After watching the delivery, we turned the television over to the news. There we were. They showed the picture Wendy had taken of the twins (I had given them approval at the news conference), and then showed a portion of the news conference itself. As I said before, the answers were all mine, but sometimes they didn't quite match the question all that well. Even with that in mind, I thought it looked pretty good. I seemed happy and confident. Just don't ask me to do it again next year.

There was one part of the conference that did upset Sandi just a bit. Early on in the questioning, someone had asked me if I had a picture of my wife. At the time I hadn't had one on me. I had, however, been carrying her drivers license. I don't even remember exactly why I had it. I put the media people off as long as I could, then, at the end of the interview, I showed them her driver's license. I really thought they just wanted to see what she looked like.

Well, there it was, right on the television screen, as big as life, for all to see, Sandi's picture. I can't recall ever meeting anyone who liked their driver's license picture. My wife was not an exception. She was temporarily (I hoped) angry with me. Luckily, there were more important things to think about. I hadn't yet been home, and didn't know just what to expect when I got there. Also, we had some planning to do as far as visitation of the babies was concerned. Sandi was still a little groggy, and very sore, so I didn't think it would be a good idea to stay a whole lot longer. We finished discussing the most important issues, saving the remainder for the following day.

I pulled myself out of the chair and got ready to go. First, however, there was something I had promised to do. I reached into my pocket and pulled out the rosary that had been given to me in the waiting room at Children's. I took time to make sure Sandi understood how important I thought it was, and then related the story of the little girl, her family and this rosary. With teary eyes, she took the rosary, and nodded her head. She had understood.

I kissed her good-bye, left the hospital and headed home, prepared to take care of whatever business might be left there yet undone.

I reached home just after 11:00. I gave Tanja a full update and asked her if she had seen us on television. She said she had been too worried to turn the news on, so I told her about the press conference.

There were numerous messages waiting for me there, much as I had suspected. Some were just from well wishes, asking no reply. Most, however, were from the media. Just about all of the local television stations and newspapers had called. There were also messages from two television networks. Some of those who had left messages had already spoken to me at the hospital, so I assumed they did not need to speak again. Just to be safe, however, I figured I would return all of the calls. Some, obviously, would have to wait until the next day. I made some notes to take with me in the morning, and then decided I should probably get some sleep.

Sleep did not come easily. Although I had been pretty well drained by the day's events, I still found my mind racing as I lay my head on the pillow. So much had happened in the past two days. So many ups and downs. I had never imagined it would be like that. I kept thinking of Megan and Shannon, picturing what they had looked like before and after surgery. More and more, I began to realize what a marvelous gift we had been given. The fate of our twin daughters was still in the hands of others. With the help of God, however, the responsibility to care for and nurture these little angels would soon be transferred over to us. We would be taking over where the doctors left off. God, I knew, would still be there with us, guiding and protecting his children.

I had promised my daughter Leanne, that she and her husband Ray could go with me to see the girls Saturday morning. Tanja also wanted to go, so it looked as though we would have a full vehicle. We had hoped to leave Sandi's two older daughters with a sitter, but they had other ideas. They knew they wouldn't be allowed in NICU yet, but they wanted to be close to their new sisters. Ray and Leanne were also bringing their three children, (my grandchildren), Sean, Nick and Melissa. So as it turned out, we required two vehicles.

We were all over the TV and radio again that morning. The three major newspapers all covered the story as well. According to the reports, the doctors had hailed the successful separation as a miracle. We didn't find any reason to disagree. I spoke with Sandi before leaving for the hospital. She had called Children's twice during the night, and spoken to the nurses on duty. Everything was okay thus far. The girls had remained stable through the night. If the news were the same at this time tomorrow, we would have cleared yet one more hurdle. I was anxious to see my little girls again, and to do whatever I could to help their healing.

The traffic was not bad on the way into the city that morning. I guess we had beaten the crowd. As we parked our vans, and headed across the street to the hospital entrance, I glanced around. I think I was half expecting someone with a television camera to jump out in front of us and start shooting. It didn't happen. When we entered the building, however, we were treated just a little differently than we had been the day before. They recognized us. The security guard even called me Mr. Fanning. I was impressed, but, at the same time, a little embarrassed. I wasn't sure if I liked the idea of being even a small celebrity. I was only a concerned father, on his way to see his critically ill children. I didn't mind the media coverage, but it didn't make us any more or less important than any other parents.

The staff in NICU also recognized us, which was good. There would need to be a lot of interfacing and we probably would end up knowing one and other fairly well. They had changed their plans on where to place Megan. Originally, she was to be located across the unit from Shannon, due to the space and equipment requirements. Now, they had moved the baby who would have been closest to Shannon over to that spot, thus allowing our girls to be no more than ten feet apart. Visiting would be much easier this way.

Before we scrubbed, I explained to the others what to expect. The twins had undergone major surgery, and were in critical but stable condition. They would still be immobilized and unconscious. The entire abdominal area would be bandaged on both girls. In addition, there would be monitors, wires and needles attached to different parts of their little bodies. It would not be a particularly pleasant sight.

They all had more or less known what to expect anyway, and had prepared themselves.

When I walked into the room where my daughters were, my emotions again kicked in. I was so very happy to be with them, but, of course, they had no idea I was even there. Just looking at them, I realized just what critical meant in their cases. They were both in open incubators, with respirators, IVs and monitors of all sorts. I thought about how lucky we were to have been living in this era. How many children like our daughters would have stood a chance of surviving just a few short years ago? Sad to say, the answer would almost certainly be none. Before all such equipment was available, there must have been many little lives cut short, many sad and lonely parents. God had been good to us.

The girls looked a little different that morning. Primarily as a result of all the anesthesia, their little bodies had swelled up. Again, I was glad Sandi had not been there to see them. They actually looked like little blow-up dolls that had been over-inflated. I knew it was temporary, but that didn't make it any easier.

Ray, Leanne and Tanja had reacted well. You could see in their eyes that each one was deeply touched. They all wanted to be with the girls, touch them, talk to them and show them that they were loved. I was happy they had come with me.

I had again brought the camera with to document the girls story. Once more, although it still didn't feel totally right, I shot some film and took some stills. When I had spoken to Sandi earlier, she had commented that Doctor Pielet might release her later in the day. I was to call back from Children's to find out what her status was.

It just also happened to be the very same day my family had planned a shower for Sandi. They had previously decided not to cancel, but rather to go ahead and have someone open the presents and someone else videotape the whole thing. When I explained to Helen that Sandi might be released that day, she asked if I thought we might be able to stop by for a few minutes on the way home. I told her I would let her know before we left Lutheran General.

I continued my visit with the twins, hoping to see some small improvement while I was there, and trying to get used to the way they looked with all of the paraphernalia hooked up. Satisfied that I had done all I could for them up to that point, I decided to check on Sandi.

I phoned Park Ridge to see if her status had changed. She said that they had agreed to release her, as long as she had someone with her for a least a few days. She was quite sore, and getting around was going to be difficult.

While we were on the phone, she told me that the media had been contacting the hospital regularly, to inquire on her condition. It appeared as though some people wanted to make sure they were not going to miss reporting on the mother of the conjoined twins leaving the hospital.

Media services at Lutheran General had offered to set-up a press conference for later that day. The plan for us was to get Sandi checked out, attend the news conference, then head for home. Otherwise, we wouldn't get any peace until every station and newspaper had interviewed the mother of the twins. One of the TV stations had also called me several times, in an attempt to obtain some footage of the girls following surgery. Children's would not, of course, allow them in. They called me, therefore, to see if I would be willing to provide footage. I guess they all knew that I had been carrying an 8mm camera around the hospital.

I hadn't been sure it would be the right thing to do, so I had told them I would get back to them. In the meantime, I had discussed it with Sandi. She hadn't been crazy about it either. After thinking about for a while, however, we had decided that I should go ahead and do it. We hadn't seen that it could do any harm, and, on the other hand, we really hadn't wanted to get the media on the wrong side. I had called them back and told them I would do it.

They sent a courier to the hospital with a blank tape, while we were visiting with Shannon and Megan. I met him in the lobby, and he waited while I made the tape. All they needed was two or three minutes of soundless footage, some of each baby. That was no problem. I filmed about one and one half minutes of each, then returned to the lobby with the tape. They were in such a rush, I really couldn't take the time to double check what I had given them.

When I got back to NICU, I realized I still had their tape in my pocket. What had I given them? I wondered. The reason they had supplied a tape in the first place, was because I had run out of my own tapes. I had told them this when they called. I had planned to take some footage that day just for us, using a tape which had previously been recorded on. When I had received the tape provided by the station, I had removed the other from the camera and stuck it in a pocket. After recording the three minutes on their tape, I had stuck it in a different pocket. Apparently, when I had rushed back down to the courier, I had reached into the wrong pocket. They were about to see a lot more than three minutes of a poorly taped men's hockey game.

I thought about what I should do. One little voice inside my head chuckled and said" do nothing." Another voice, however, proved to be a little stronger. This one said "be responsible, call them." The stronger voice won. I called, told them what had happened and apologized. They contacted the courier immediately and had him make a U turn. A few minutes later, he pulled up in front of the hospital, rapidly exchanged the tapes and then sped off as if the KGB were on his tail. "Boy," I thought. All this for three minutes of film.

When I got back to NICU, I still didn't feel right. Our babies were going to be shown on TV, in critical condition, with all the medical paraphernalia attached and operating. Was it really the right thing to do? I didn't think there was a yes or no answer. Looking at it one way, it seemed wrong. Looking at it another, however, we were going to be providing a lot of people with what they wanted. There were many interested and caring people who would never be able to actually see the twins in person. As a matter of fact, there were friends and relatives who would not be able to see our home videos. They deserved an update also. It began to look like we had done the right thing.

I went to scrub, so I could again touch my daughters. First, however, I loaded the tape of the hockey game into the camera. We had said there would be no exclusives. I needed to film another three minutes to provide to the other stations.

We finished our visit with Shannon and Megan, then started out for Park Ridge. Leanne and Ray had also planned to visit Sandi that day, so they followed us from one hospital to the other.

The atmosphere at Lutheran General was great. It wasn't really circus like, but everyone was happy and positive; and there were a lot of people there to be that way. It seemed as though everyone who had anything to do with Sandi or the twins was there.

Doctor Pielet had accomplished his goal, he had delivered the babies six weeks premature, yet basically fully developed. Thanks to him and his staff, our girls had gotten a real good shot at making it. He was more jovial than I had remembered seeing him, and more talkative.

It seemed everyone there was also talkative. Mostly, of course, about the twins, but about other things as well. The media, for instance, was a fairly popular topic. At one point, someone made a statement that "if the media was willing to wait for hours to catch the mother checking out of the hospital, how long would they wait to catch her visiting the twins for the first time." When I heard that, I decided to speak to Sandi about it. I was afraid they might be correct. Someone would be waiting for her at Children's later that evening.

Sandi and I discussed the issue alone, as soon as we got a chance. We decided it would be better if we did not go back to see the twins that evening, but rather, went directly home. We would phone Children's to make sure the girls were okay, and then head into Chicago very early Sunday morning. It was quite unlikely there would be anyone still waiting between 2:00 and 5:00 in the morning.

The press conference with Sandi and Doctor Pielet had now been set up for 2:00 that afternoon. I filled them in on what sort of questions had been asked at my conference the previous day. Since all of the stations kept re-using the same two or three minutes, I thought they might like to know what I was asked and how I responded during the remaining twelve or thirteen.

Shortly before 2:00, we were notified that one of the media representatives would be delayed. They asked us if we would postpone the conference until 2:30. We agreed, the extra half hour wait did not seem to present a large inconvenience.

When everyone had arrived, we were ushered down to the auditorium. By that time, I must have seemed pretty sure of myself in regards to questions from the media. One of the doctors commented that I was becoming a real celebrity and he wondered if one of the television stations might have asked me to do a special yet. I couldn't help myself, it seemed like as good a time as any to try one of my "special" answers. "As a matter of fact," I replied in a serious manner, "yes they have. They want me to star in a television movie with Tonya Harding."

The doctor hesitated for a couple of seconds, then looked

at me and smiled.

The press conference wasn't a lot different than the one I had been involved in the previous day. There were some of the same questions. They were, however, worded differently so as to be more appropriate for the mother; and there were a couple of new ones.

Sandi handled herself quite well, as I had known she would, answering all of the questions posed to her calmly and proficiently. She showed just enough of her emotions to make everyone understand that what she had been through thus far, had been no picnic.

Doctor Pielet also got a chance to answer a couple of questions, and handled them with professional ease.

The conference was followed, as before, by some informal conversation. One of the newspapers used the time to interview us for a special article, while other reporters talked with some of the family members who were present. Amanda ended up getting an interview with a reporter, who promised her it would be on TV later that evening.

A representative of one of the television stations asked, at that time, if I had any more pictures or footage they could use. I said "as a matter of fact, I do, but you'll have to share it." I tossed them the tape, explained about needing to ignore the hockey game portion and requested that they promise to return it to me.

They agreed and asked if all of the stations could use it. I said "all but channel 7, they have their own copy."

The mood, as I said, was basically a happy one. We had much to be happy and thankful for.

The conversation ended pleasantly, and we finished the task of checking Sandi out of the hospital. As might have been expected, there was some emotion involved in her leaving. She had made many friends during her four and one half week stay at Lutheran General. While everyone was happy for her and the girls, there would be a little piece of their lives missing after she had gone. Amidst hugs and tears, I gently pushed her wheel chair to the front exit. It was time to go.

I had told Sandi previously about the shower that was being held for her. Although she was not very mobile and certainly did not feel like visiting, she wanted to stop by on the way home. It was already getting late, but Helen's house was not far out of the way. It wouldn't hurt to drop in for a few minutes.

We got into our van. Together again after too many weeks. It didn't take long for our thoughts to turn to the children who could not be with us. Megan and Shannon wouldn't have known the difference right then, but as short as their lives had been thus far, they were already dearly missed and greatly loved.

The atmosphere at Lutheran General had been a happy one and had served to take our minds off of the dangers that still lay ahead. Once we were on the road, however, it had been only natural for us to focus back on the twins. We knew only too well that they had a long way to go to recovery. Showing our happiness over the success experienced thus far was alright, but this was still a very serious situation. We would continue to pray to God, hope for the best outcome, and do everything within our power to help get our babies healthy and strong.

We stopped briefly at the shower. It was just winding down when we arrived, which was fine. We hadn't planned on staying long anyway. To say that everyone their was glad to see Sandi would have been an understatement. Many of those present had not seen her for more than five months. Some, I think, were still a little bit in awe over the media coverage. Everyone was, however, sincerely happy for the twins success thus far, and very hopeful for the future.

There were many wonderful and useful gifts brought there by the attendees, but they were overshadowed by the great support shown us by friends and family.

We left my sister's house and headed for what we hoped would be the quiet warmth of our own home.

When we arrived, we were both very tired. Sandi could barely move and was extremely sore. Our plan was to answer messages, call the hospital to check on the twins and then go to bed. Since the media had been brought up to date just a few hours earlier, they shouldn't have to bother us.

There turned out to be a couple of messages from television stations and another from a newspaper. One station wanted to do a short spot with the both of us within the next day or two. The newspaper needed additional information for an article. The third message was actually from a national network wanting approval to use the videotape we had supplied to one of the local stations. I managed to get through to the network and give them our approval. It was too late to reach the others, so I made a note to call them the following day.

We now had a list of phone messages over two pages long. These were from people other than relatives or close friends. Some of them were from strangers, wishing us the best of luck. Most, however, were from newspapers and television stations, local and out of state. They all wanted more information, more film or more pictures. We had already made up our minds to be accommodating, but squeezing in all of these return phone calls was getting difficult to accomplish. We would just do the best we could.

We called the hospital to check on the twins. They had previously arranged it so that when we called, we could speak directly with the nurses in charge of the girls. Because of their conditions, they each had their own nurse and were never left unattended, day or night. That was comforting. Even more so, however, was the knowledge and caring attitude shown by these nurses. They were professional, they knew their stuff and they truly cared.

Sandi had already called the girls room a good number of times. She was yet to be there personally, but some of the nurses could already recognize her voice.

The twins were fine. There had been no change in their general condition or status. The nurses on duty told Sandi that when we visited in the morning, someone would explain all of the equipment, it's various functions and just what the different fluids were going into and coming out of both girls. That pleased Sandi. She had majored in Biology and at one time, planned on entering the medical field. She, most likely, would more easily understand what it was all about.

We got to bed fairly early, managed to actually catch some sleep, then rose long before daybreak, in an attempt to have a quiet, private visit with the twins.

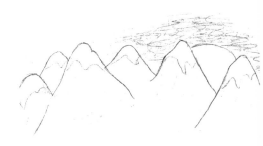

CHAPTER 13

Clearing Hurdles

It was early in the morning when we arrived at Children's. Even from the eighth floor window, the warm rays of the spring sun had not yet reached out across the blue-green surface of Lake Michigan. To some, it must have seemed like a typical morning for that time of the year. To my wife, however, there wasn't anything typical about it. She was going to see her twin daughters for the first time following their major surgery. She was understandably nervous and, though I did my best to calm and comfort her, only after she had touched and kissed each baby, would she relax at all.

I had tried to prepare Sandi by reminding her of what the nurses had told us to expect. The babies would be heavily sedated, somewhat physically restrained and attached to all sorts of equipment. While they would still be beautiful, the sight of them in such condition, might be rather upsetting.

I had explained that both girls were "puffed up" or swollen. I had not, however, been able to properly relate the severity of the swelling. Sandi might have known about what to expect, she just hadn't realized it would be so severe. As she was re-united with our newborn daughters, now separated by more than ten feet, she wept.

We continued our visit. As Sandi grew more accustomed to the way the girls looked, she began to ask questions about the equipment and the different drugs used.

That first visit was emotionally touching, but also rather quiet and private. I was glad to get it over with, as I had been worried about what Sandi's initial reaction might be. I was also, however, encouraged by the healthy, positive

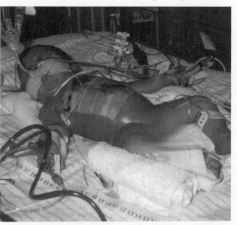

atmosphere that was present. I felt a little better about leaving the twins that day.

It was early Sunday afternoon when we returned home from the visit. Sandi's mood was of resolve and res

After separation surgery, the girls were swollen, heavily sedated and in extremely critical condition. Seeing them this way brought tears to my eyes; but, at least now the healing could begin.

ponsibility. Just as she had done every-thing in her power

to protect and nurture the twins in her womb, she was now resolved to do whatever necessary to protect their health and improve their chances for survival in the outside world. We talked about it a lot during the drive from Chicago. Besides continued prayer, their was only so much we could do. The doctors and nurses certainly seemed to have things well in hand. To Sandi, however, being with the twins as much as possible, and keeping them in our thoughts when we weren't with them, was, at least, a good start.

I agreed with her. I was still working, so I would only be able to get down to see them four or five times a week, and sometimes maybe only three. Sandi, on the other hand, would be there every day.

Sandi hoped that, with these daily visits, she could let the girls know she was there, and also learn everything she could from the doctors and nurses. If she ever had to make a split second medical decision concerning the twins, she would be prepared.

The first two days had seemed to be creeping by. The doctors had said that if the girls got through the weekend okay, then one more hurdle would be out of the way. By the time we left on Sunday, they admitted that we had indeed successfully passed that critical forty-eight hour period.

We had assumed that we would be able to rest a little easier once the weekend had passed. It wasn't so, however. The girls were still both in critical condition, although they remained stable. The seriousness of the surgery and the inability to completely identify the biliary tract in either baby, were still reasons for major concern. In addition,

Megan's swelling was not decreasing as quickly as Shannon's. She was holding fluid, particularly in the area of the head.

The week was drawing to a close. The girls had begun to open their eyes on occasion, and to move limbs in a limited manner, but progress seemed slow. Sandi and I wondered if we were expecting too much too soon. The doctors had been very guarded when asked about the twins' condition. Basically, all they would say was that the girls were doing about as expected. It was tough to be with our babies so much and have them not even know we were around.

I couldn't erase some of the statistics that just kept popping back into my head. One of the most disconcerting, was that regarding the percentage of cases where separation was completely successful.

There was one set of twins, joined similarly to ours, that had been successfully separated. But, even with those lovely girls, there had been permanent problems. Both girls had undergone colostomies and were incontinent. At least, though, they were alive, healthy and loved. So many of the other sets of conjoined twins, about which we had read or heard, had not been so lucky. I would do my best to keep those other sets of twins out of my mind.

Life away from Children's Memorial continued to be quite busy. There were only so many hours in each day and most of them were being spent either with the girls or doing something related to their hospital stay. There were a couple of more interviews for newspapers, and one TV station had asked us to do a special update for Easter.

Since the girls had been slowly improving, we had agreed to their request. The idea of the update was to show

how it was to be a special Easter for our family. Sandi and I managed to change the theme just a little. As far as we were concerned, it was a Thanksgiving Easter. That's how it ended up coming across on television. Everyone thought it went very well. They even managed to get a shot of the special painting and fish stenciling we had done in the girls room. As the reporter said "their room is ready and waiting." We agreed.

That first week was Holy Week for most Christians. Between Sandi being at the hospital most of the time, and me splitting a good portion of my time between work and the hospital, we had little opportunity to attend Holy Week services. On the way to visit the girls Good Friday, I found myself apologizing to God. We were asking an awful lot from him, I felt guilty about not showing more respect for his son.

Sandi said she believed God would understand. She was, apparently, correct. That day, the doctors upgraded both girls' conditions from critical to serious. This wasn't due to any sudden, drastic change for the better, but rather, the overall trend of improvement seen during that week. Whatever the reason, we were very happy. It looked like the twins had cleared that important seven to ten day hurdle. Serious sure sounded a lot better than critical.

In addition to phone calls from TV stations wanting updates, we continued to get the odd special request. One such request came from a local TV station. It just happened to be one that is seen all over North America by cable or satellite. I had received the call that Friday, They asked me if I would be interested in appearing live at 10:00 P.M. that Saturday as a "Newsmaker." I talked it over with Sandi, then called them back and said yes.

Holy Saturday, we had already visited the twins prior to heading for the station's Chicago studio. They had shown some more improvement. In fact, both girls had been extubated. In hospital terms, that meant the doctors had removed their oxygen tubes. We felt good about their continuing positive reports, even if the progress was not as rapid as we had hoped for.

We arrived at the studio around 9:30. Once we got past the security desk, everyone was very friendly and helpful. We were introduced to all the news people, and they really seemed interested in the girls. They were also, very happy to see that Sandi had made the trip with me. As a matter of fact, since we were both there, and they only had room to interview one person, they asked if she would go on instead of me. I didn't mind all that much, after all, she was the mom. She looked at it somewhat differently. She said that they had asked for me, and I should be the one going on the air. I believe she actually thought it would be unfair to me if she appeared, and that I might feel bad. In any case, I went on as the "Newsmaker of The Week." The station didn't mind, as long as they had one of us.

The spot was only about two minutes long, and I was live. Based on those two facts, I asked for some idea of what questions would be asked of me. I was given four different questions they said might be asked. It was over quickly, and everyone commented on how well they thought I had handled myself. That was pretty impressive, I thought, especially since none of the questions asked of me was one of the four they had provided prior to the interview.

The following day was Easter Sunday. We had planned to spend a good portion of it with the twins. Sandi had continued to call and talk to their nurses each night, or any other time we were away from them for more than a few hours. She had been unable to get through most of that night. She had finally reached the girls room at around 4:30 in the morning. We almost wished she hadn't.

Megan had gone through a bad night. A couple of hours earlier she had experienced a seizure. They were not sure what had caused it, but she was immediately placed on regular doses of Phenobarbital and Dilantin. It was also necessary for them to re-intubate her. It was a step backwards.

We rushed to the hospital. There wasn't much we could do, but we wanted to be with her as soon as possible anyway. We hoped that by now, they were both able to sense our presence. In the van, on our way there we again said a special prayer.

The neonatal unit seemed more subdued than normal when we arrived. In fact, the whole hospital seemed a lot quieter. We were surprised that this would be so on Easter Sunday.

In the girls room, Megan was a sad sight. She was, once more completely immobile, with a breathing tube down her throat. We had known better than to get our hopes up too high because of the progress we had seen thus far. That didn't matter. She had been better and now she was worse. It was our first setback, and it was very painful.

We attempted to find out just what this seizure meant.

Did it indicate other problems? Were there likely to be more seizures? How long would it be until we would know for sure if she was going to be okay? Obviously, the answers weren't there. We would just have to wait.

The Easter Bunny had made a visit to NICU and left little stuffed animals for the girls. Obviously, however, it was not as happy a day as we had planned for. We still had an awful lot to be thankful for, and tried to remember that.

The following day, Megan was given an EEG and a CAT scan. Since she had retained fluid, the doctors thought she might have some on the brain. The other possibility they wanted to check on, was the bursting of a blood vessel. Either one could have caused her seizure. That same day, Sandi was allowed to hold both her little angels, one in each arm. She cried.

The test results came back apparently negative. There did not seem to be any fluid build-up. There was, however, a possibility that a small vessel had indeed burst, but they couldn't say for sure. The EEG had also shown Megan was still experiencing silent seizures. In other words, they detected brain wave patterns that indicated visible seizures would be occurring if she had not been taking the prescribed drugs.

The doctors tried not to appear negative when they made their explanations to us. One of the last statements they made was actually fairly positive. They said that the seizures could have been one-time spontaneous. They could have been caused by the sudden loss of body fluids.

Megan had been receiving medication to help her get rid of some of the excess fluid. It was possible that the medication had been responsible for such a sudden fluid loss; thus triggering the seizure. We really hoped that this had been the case.

The girls had now passed the magical tenth day. With Megan's set back, it hardly seemed significant. There were, however, some real positive things to consider.

One of the key elements in evaluating the twins' progress, was the ability of their bodies to process and dispose of food. This would eventually tell the doctors if the kidneys, liver, bowel, stomach and bladder were functioning; and if the girls biliary tracts were complete and operational. The beginning of what we would consider normal body functions would turn out to be events of significant importance.

The first of the functions to take place was urination. Catheters had been inserted into the bladders of both girls. These were attached by means of tubing, to plastic bags. It didn't take long for the twins to begin filling the bags. Both were urinating well within the first twenty-four hours. There seemed to be no kidney or bladder problems.

The biliary tract was a different issue. The girls had OG tubes inserted through their mouths and into the stomachs. The tubes drew out the contents of the stomach. This was initially dark green bile. As they healed, should everything be alright inside, this fluid would change in color to greenish yellow and then, finally, yellow.

Since the girls were being fed intravenously, the kidneys had been doing most of the work, processing the liquid diet. Once they started having mom's milk fed directly into their stomachs, however, attention was turned toward another bodily function, the bowel movement. The doctors had spent a lot of time on the girls' bowels. They were anxious to see how well their handy work had turned out.

The girls were into their second week of hospitalization, and had been given NG tubes for feeding. Attempts were now being made to feed Shannon by bottle, while Megan was still basically "out of it" most of the time due to the drugs she was being given.

We worried about her greatly. She was the larger of the two, probably outweighing her sister by at least twelve ounces at birth. That doesn't sound like a lot, but when you figure that their combined weight had been seven pounds twelve ounces, you get a better picture of just how much larger she was.

Because of the size difference, everyone had been more concerned about Shannon. She was so small, could she pull through this?

Inside their mother's womb, Shannon had been the feisty one. She had been more active than her larger sister and more easily agitated. Now, outside the comfort of her mother's protection, she was still feisty. She seemed to be telling everyone that size had nothing to do with toughness. Some of the staff members thought she was doing surprisingly well, and told us so. Did that mean she was out of the woods? No, apparently it was much too early for that.

If it were too early for Shannon to be out of danger, then what about Megan? She had fallen significantly behind her sister. Would she catch up? and what about the seizures! Day after day these questions were there, waiting for answers. We wondered just when we would ever be holding our girls as healthy happy babies.

Sandi and I spent a lot of our time just talking about the girls. We knew we had good reason to be concerned, but remembering what the doctors had told us, perhaps we were being too impatient. They had, after all, said that hospital recovery would be four to five weeks. It had, at that time, been just over two. There was a lot of healing to be done. It was true that babies have their own recuperative powers, far superior to those of adults, but maybe it was just too early for those powers to have done the job. The doctors knew what they were doing, and God certainly knew what he was doing as well. We would just have to be patient, while doing whatever we could to help them heal.

The twins had been receiving milk by tube for a couple of days. It would only be a matter of time before we knew if the bowels were operating properly. We didn't realize how closely the doctors were watching for this, until the first movement took place.

Doctor Moss had just completed his rounds, when we entered the girls' room. The nurse, as always, was helpful and friendly. She had something special, however, to tell us this time. Shannon had her first bowel movement. We were extremely happy to here this.

According to the nurse, Doctor Moss had been even happier than Sandi and I. She said she really thought he was going to dance a jig. The same reaction apparently took place following Megan's first movement. This whole incident certainly confirmed the criticality of the issue concerning the biliary tracts and bowels. The doctors had been more concerned than we thought, that was certain. Sandi and I had been right to be so worried, maybe now we could relax just a little.

The third week offered us another opportunity to test our emotional strength. It started well, with notable progress being made by both girls. Then, on Wednesday, April 12th, Shannon had her own set-back. She vomited green. This was a sign of possible bowel obstruction. There was significant concern on the part of the entire staff. A bowel obstruction would mean surgery was needed, and needed soon. Shannon still weighed well under four pounds, and had not yet recuperated from the initial surgery. Chances of her surviving another serious surgical procedure at this time would be small. We waited for the radiology report, and we prayed.

The test results showed that the possibility of an obstruction certainly did exist, they were not, however, conclusive. Close monitoring of the situation would be necessary, until they were sure the bowels were functioning properly. The lack of regular bowel movements, or the "throwing up" of bile would be an indication of an obstruction. Unfortunately, we knew what we would have to do, and we were getting used to it. We would have to wait.

The following day, Megan received another ultrasound of the head. The purpose was to help determine if hemorrhage had occurred in conjunction with her earlier seizure. The results, happily, showed no evidence of hemorrhage. The doctors commented that it was looking more like the seizure had been spontaneous. They stated that, many times a child will have one such seizure, and never experience another. They would, however, be keeping her on anti-seizure medication for a least a couple of additional months. Once she returned home, we would have to wean her from it gradually. The part about her returning home sure sounded good.

The next day, it was Megan who again gave us reason for concern. The nurses noticed that fluid was leaking from her central line, (the tube inserted into her chest, through which initial feeding had taken place). It was necessary for her to have yet another radiograph.

The test results revealed what appeared to be a clot in her vein. Our own hearts stopped for a second when we heard this. Megan could not afford problems which would in any way affect her heart. She had been diagnosed earlier, as having a heart murmur. There was actually a small hole in her heart. The doctors had said she may require surgery later on. They had told us it was difficult to tell in premature babies just what the outcome might be.

This type of clot, as it turned out, was not all that uncommon with central lines. When such a line remained in place for a period of time, this often occurred. They were able to clean the chest area and the insertion point. They then applied a fluid to dissolve the clot. The whole process was completed that same day.

We had learned by this time, that, Doctor Raffensperger, besides being more experienced than the other doctors, was also more of an aggressive risk-taker. The situation with Megan's central line was all he needed to order the lines removed from both girls permanently. According to him, they should be feeding, through the mouth, taking as much of mom's milk as possible anyway. Both twins were also receiving some medication through these lines, so the staff would just have to make sure they came up with something which could be administered orally. That day, he interrupted our visit and asked us to leave the room while surgery was performed. As we waited outside the unit, he removed both central lines.

The girls began doing very well without their central lines. They both continued to gradually improve. The amount of mother's milk being consumed by each slowly increased. The majority of the feeding was still being done orally, through NG tubes. Shannon began however, to take some milk by bottle, and a little directly from her mother. Megan, on the other hand, was getting hers almost strictly through the tube.

The third week of recovery passed without any more significant happenings. We had begun the all important fourth week. Both girls were now having regular, but loose, bowel movements. Sandi had become somewhat persistent in asking the doctors about taking the twins home. We realized that we, as parents, would be taking on a huge task. It would be necessary for us to provide the same type of care at home, as the girls were getting in the hospital. To a large degree, we would be their new nurses. We believed we could handle the situation with minimal difficulty. Sandi had watched and assisted the nurses at every opportunity. She would be able to perform all of the necessary functions. She had even gotten certified by the hospital for Infant Resuscitation. She was ready.

There was a significant advantage to taking care of the babies here at the hospital, as opposed to providing the care at home. There were numerous pieces of equipment, especially monitors, which aided greatly in determining whether or not everything was alright at any given time. We had spent a lot of time watching the various monitors, and worrying when things like the breathing rate or heart rate changed unexpectedly. While I would be thrilled to take our daughters home, I realized it could also put us in a rather scary situation.

Doctor Raffensperger was eager to have us take the girls home as well. "When they get to four pounds each, take them home," he said. "I want them out of here by their one month birthday."

Doctor Moss had been a little more reserved. He didn't want to see us take them home, then have to bring them back in a few days or weeks. His answer had basically been, "we'll see."

We realized that both doctors had the girls' best interests in mind, they just looked at the situation from two slightly different perspectives. With some luck, and a little more help from the guy up above, we would be taking our daughters home the following weekend. Only, however, if both the doctors agreed.

The remainder of the week seemed to pass fairly quickly. We were assured that, although still attached and operational, the monitors were no longer required. By Wednesday, they both weighed in at over four pounds. No additional problems had occurred with either girl. On Thursday, April 21st, we were told that we could take our babies home the next day.

It had all seemed to happen so fast. One day we were still worried that they might not make it, the next thing we knew, they were coming home.

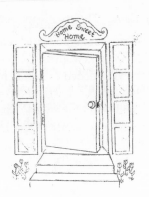

CHAPTER 14

Going Home

The media had been following the girls progress rather closely. Since we had agreed that the hospital could release statements on upgrades and progress, we were no longer getting all that many calls at home. That was good, because Sandi and I were quite busy those last days. The fewer calls the better.

Preparing for the girls at home was, actually, a big deal. The atmosphere at the hospital was clean, quiet and controlled. There were a lot of people living at our house, and we also did get a good number of regular visitors. There would have to be changes, and everyone would have to know just what was ahead. One of the biggest problems we foresaw, was that of people wanting to touch or hold the twins. The hospital environment was sterile. The girls would be more susceptible to germs at home. Everyone was just going to have follow our "rules."

We were contacted by Robin, another hospital media

services representative, who wanted to discuss the issue of the media and our girls' release. All of the stations and newspapers wanted to have someone there when the girls left. We needed to decide how and where we would see the press. Since we would be on our way out, and the girls would be with us, we would most likely be able to keep the whole thing pretty short. It was agreed to, therefore, that questions could be asked while we were in the lobby, and heading for the front doors. If that was not enough time for some of them, we were sure they would contact us at home.

The morning of April 22nd came, and we were excited. It was hard to believe it was really happening, we were taking our little angels home.

The doctors had asked us to come in early. There were a number of items they needed to go over with us. They also had some questions to ask us regarding care of the twins. Sandi and I had the feeling that, if they determined, by our answers, that we would not be able to handle some of the situations that could arise, we would not be allowed to take the twins out of the hospital at that time. I wasn't too worried. Sandi had proven to me that she was fully capable of taking care of the girls. Whatever I could do to assist, would be a bonus.

That morning, even the drive to Chicago was filled with excitement, and it wasn't the scenery that caused it. Our little twins were going to join the rest of the family. To the many people who had hoped, prayed and waited for that day, it was indeed special.

Sandi had prepared everything we would need to take with us. It had been loaded in the van and double checked long before we left home. There were all of the necessary baby items; including, two little outfits and two very nice car seats. All were gifts from the baby shower.

We had thought that Megan and Shannon, being so small, would probably swim in the clothes and be almost lost in the seats. Size, however, didn't matter, four pounds or forty, they were going with us that day.

They would be leaving the safe solitude of the hospital room for the more hectic, less technically supportive atmosphere of their nursery at home. We hoped the change would only temporarily prove unsettling. We believed the support we could supply from the heart and the soul would at least match what they had previously received from monitors and other electronic equipment.

We arrived at the hospital at around noon. Just about everyone there recognized us and had a smile or a good word.

Upon entering NICU, we were directed to a quiet room to meet with Doctor Moss. This meeting, as it turned out, showed more than any other event had, just how he cared about our girls. His eyes lit up when he spoke of the progress each had made. At the same time, he expressed real concern when he spoke of the questions and issues still unresolved.

Neither baby was feeding well from the bottle; nor were they able to regularly take milk directly from their mother. This made tube feeding necessary. Doctor Moss went over this with us, although Sandi had already shown the nurses that she knew exactly how to insert the tube, and how to make sure it had been done properly.

The doctor then went on to describe all of the medication the girls were receiving. He explained what each one was for, how much was to be given, and when. Of course, Sandi also knew how the medication was to given. She had watched and assisted many times.

The next thing on the doctors list, was an explanation of caloric intake. This included a formula for determining how many calories should be provided each feeding and each day. This was translated into amounts of milk. In addition, it was necessary for him to explain how much weight increase these calories should represent. We would need a baby scale which read in grams, as it would be extremely important to monitor the babies' weights daily. He explained to us that no weight gain for one day, or maybe even two days, at a time was okay; but should either baby show the same weight for more than two consecutive days, or should they lose any weight, we would need to bring them back to the hospital right away. This situation would be an indication of either a feeding problem and/or a bowel problem. While this whole issue worried us a good deal, it was not going to make us change our minds about taking them home. They were going with us that same day.

Doctor Moss finished our meeting by explaining what we should look for with the girls. This included the issues regarding how to tell when they were ill, how to determine when something wasn't right and when to call Children's or rush the twins to emergency. The two scariest issues were that regarding Megan's heart, and that of Shannon's possible bowel problem. I cringed when he repeated the statement, "if they vomit green, call us immediately," several times.

Just as we thought our meeting was over, Doctor Moss turned and said, rather seriously, "there's one more thing." Immediately, I thought "oh no! What didn't he tell us now?" He handed us a piece of paper and said "this is my new address in New Mexico, I'll be leaving in a few weeks. Promise me you will put me on your Christmas list and send me pictures of the twins."

This was an easy one for us to answer. We both said "no problem at all Doctor." He smiled, and we smiled back.

Once the meeting had been completed, we all headed back to the girls room. Robin was there with John, the hospital photographer. They wanted to get a few shots for their own paper. Doctor Moss had his camera as well. We made sure at least one picture was taken of him holding both girls. Sandi commented that she hoped the reflection off of his glistening eyes would not spoil the picture. I just smiled. We had gotten a little better idea, that day, of why he had been so conservative about letting the girls leave. He really cared.

If we had thought leaving the hospital with our daughters would be easy, we had been mistaken. Nevermind the fact that, as Robin had told us, there were dozens of people waiting for us downstairs; we still had a lot of unfinished hospital business. We had yet to meet with one of the certified nurses, to discuss all of the details regarding caring for the babies at home. These were still very small, premature babies who had undergone major surgery. The hospital and all the medical staff wanted to be sure we were given all the information we needed to provide for them properly.

Completing the official documentation end of the business should have been simple. But, for some reason, we ended up trying to check Megan out twice. It turned out to be a paperwork error only, and not the fact that they looked so much alike. Since a couple of the nurses had commented on wanting to keep Shannon, we did, jokingly, blame it on them.

In order to check the girls out, it was necessary for us to go down to the cashier's office on the ground floor. The main hospital elevators opened facing the lobby on the same floor. This, of course, was where all of the reporters were waiting. The nurses decided that, since I would almost certainly be recognized once I stepped out of the elevator, they would take me down through the staff elevator.

This idea worked well. From the cashier's desk, I could look down the hall and see the lobby. It was packed with reporters, photographers and interested bystanders.

One of the security guards stood next to us as I took care of the paperwork. While I was busy signing in all the right places, another guard walked up to us. Addressing the first guard, he said " what the heck is going on anyway? Do we have royalty here or what?" I didn't hear the response, but I'm sure some explanation was given. From the way most people had acted, I had assumed that everyone at the hospital was aware of who we were. It was actually a little refreshing to see someone who didn't know about us.

I still had mixed feelings about being in the limelight. I didn't mind the reporters and the cameras for short periods of time. I knew the enormous amount of interest shown would quickly decrease as the opportunity to sensationalize our situation dwindled. The media would go with whatever was hot. On the other hand, however, it did bother me that some of our comments had been taken out of context. It hadn't been enough to make us look bad or stupid, but had changed our story just a little. Everyone who was watching, listening or reading, was not getting the whole picture.

I finished with the cashier and returned to NICU. There were still a number of nurses, doctors and various other staffers, who wanted to say good-bye. We didn't mind so much, they had all been very good to us and our babies.

We took more pictures and shot a little footage with the 8 mm. There were some emotional good-byes said, then we were ready to head downstairs.

It's difficult to explain how it felt just passing through the large double doors of NICU with our daughters. There had been times when I seriously wondered if it would ever happen. I had never experienced anything like it with any of my other children. My emotions had been rocked, and sometimes even battered, during the previous few months. This homecoming was adding yet another chapter to the story. I had a hard time holding back the tears of joy.

We had again decided to use the staff elevator. As before, there was no one waiting for us when the doors opened. This turned out to be even more beneficial. Not only did it give us the opportunity to see them coming and try to prepare, but it also allowed Sandi to say a special good-bye to someone.

Throughout the girls' stay in NICU, there was one little boy, within a few feet of them, but behind a wall made mostly of glass. His name was Matthew O'Brien, and his room was kept even more sterile than that of the twins.

Sandi had hoped to see his mother before we left, to say good-bye, wish her luck, and pass on to her the rosary she had used in praying for the lives and health of our daughters. This was the same rosary that had been passed on to me by the family who shared the waiting room with us the day of the surgery.

Mrs. O'Brien just happened to be outside the elevator doors. Sandi wasted no time in taking care of her special good-bye. She gave her the rosary and our best wishes, then tearfully returned to my side.

The crowd recognized us while we were still in the hallway. They descended upon us within seconds.

Sandi leaned over to me and said "if they ask a stupid question like 'your daughters have finally been released from the hospital. What are you going to do now?', what will we say?" I looked at her for a second or two, then we both said together, "We're going to Disneyworld."

It was good to know that Sandi and I still thought alike. Not only that, but even after all of the difficult times we had recently see, we were both able to maintain our sense of humor.

We turned back to the reporters and began addressing their questions. It was actually a fairly short interview. They couldn't think of a lot of things they hadn't already asked. I believe their main goal was to get footage of the twins. We didn't mind. This was still a happy story, and the girls were beautiful. Besides, we knew that nobody would be able to misquote anything Shannon or Megan had to say.

When the questions had died down, I left the group so that I could pull our van up to the front door.

They had a loading area marked in front of the hospital. When I got there, however, it was blocked by another vehicle. Since we would only be a few minutes, I thought it might be alright if I just pulled up behind the other car. As I got out of the van, I found out I had been wrong.

A gentleman, obviously employed by the hospital, immediately confronted me. "What do you think you're doing?" he asked. "You can't park there."

"I'm sorry," I replied. "Where should I park?"

"Up there," he said, pointing to the area just in front of the other car.

I didn't take the time to explain that, when I arrived, I couldn't get to that particular spot. I just said "okay", and moved the van.

In the meantime, another security guard came out to talk to the gentleman who had made me move. They were both waiting for me when I got out of my van.

"I'm sorry Mr. Fanning," said the first gentleman. "I didn't know it was you. I was just doing what I normally would have done."

I was glad he gave me the opportunity to reply. I smiled at him and said, "don't apologize, you did the right thing. I'm just another visitor here, no better or worse than anyone else. I don't expect to be treated differently."

He seemed relieved, but continued to act as though there

was something special about us. He cleared a path for Sandi and the girls, and made sure all the other traffic was held up. I even had some difficulty loading all of our stuff into the van without him helping.

Since everybody likes being treated special once in a while, I decided these few minutes wouldn't hurt. As it turned out, he actually ended up being somewhat helpful by providing another obstacle for people to pass in order to ask additional questions.

Once the van was loaded, we said good-bye to the nurses who had accompanied us out through the hospital front doors.

These three ladies represented the eight or ten nurses who had regularly taken care of our daughters. It was impossible for us to leave with dry eyes. None of the ladies attempted to hold back the tears. It was a very emotional and extremely touching good-bye. I myself, managed to keep my outward display to a little moisture around the surface of my eyes. Inwardly, however, my heart was filled thankfulness, love and admiration for those who had so diligently and lovingly cared for our daughters.

With our good-byes complete, it was time to go. Once inside, I rolled down the van window to address one final question. The cameras continued to roll, as we headed away from Children's Memorial, toward the familiar warmth of our own home.

The drive to Naperville was long. The rush hour had just begun and traffic was heavy. We didn't really mind much though. The girls were with us, and they were resting peacefully.

Once we got home, I felt like I never wanted to leave.

The babies were alright for now, and we were all tired out from the day's excitement. Somehow, though, I had a feeling that we were only just starting another chapter in our own amazing adventure. I hoped and prayed that this one would be the happiest, least erratic thus far.

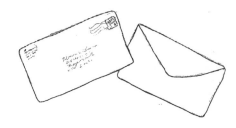

CHAPTER 15

Major Support

It wasn't long after the girls' surgery, that the support being received increased. I don't just mean financial. Yes, there was a little of that. It was the other types of support, however, that added so much to this story.

To begin with, there was a great amount of what I would call physical support. That is, people offering to perform various functions to help us out during this period. This included: free baby-sitting for Sandi's two older daughters, cooking of complete dinners, providing transportation, helping with household or yard chores, providing a listening ear, giving Sandi and I a free "get-away," knitting, stitching or sewing all sorts of baby things and many more miscellaneous activities. Friends, relatives and acquaintances were calling regularly to see how they could be of assistance. We were overwhelmed and flattered.

Sandi and I tried our best to accept only that which we really needed. We didn't want to hurt anyone's feelings, so each offer was weighed individually. It was not a simple task. The whole issue made us rather uncomfortable. It was plain to see that a family in our situation, could easily take advantage of well-wishers offering assistance. It would be all too simple.

The specific incidences of physical support were many indeed. There were a few, however, that stood out more than the others.

The parish to which we belong, Saint Margaret Mary, provides many support services to parishioners and community members. Not the least of these involves volunteers cooking and delivering full dinners to families in hard time, or crisis situations. For two months, we received three large, excellent dinners each week. These meals included everything, and were delivered to us at a pre-arranged time and day. In addition, some friends also provided dinners at least once a week, during the same period. All of this helped enormously, as we had little or no time to prepare such meals ourselves.

When it came to baby supplies, we really were in need. Because we had been so concerned about the outcome of the surgery, we had pretty much stayed away from shopping. There was much we would need.

We began, therefore, to take some people up on their offers. Sandi's friend Terry had a crib, a cradle and a swing she had thought we might be able to use. We decide she had been right. We used these items to have the girls' room all ready for them when they got home.

There were many people also offering baby clothes and other small items. We even ended getting some clothes back, which had been used by Sandi for her youngest, then by my daughter and eventually by my niece Brenda. Wherever they came from, we were glad for the offers.

Many people believe that it is possible for the family to benefit financially from a situation such as ours. I suppose that it could be, but I would doubt that such a thought would very often be on that families minds. Whoever, God forbid, may find themselves in a similar situation, with the lives of not one, but two of their children hanging in the balance, will know that the financial aspects mean absolutely nothing. That is, of course, unless actual cash is required in order to have necessary medical treatment provided. This was not the case with us.

The issue of money or insurance was never brought up by either Sandi or I, and we certainly never asked for any sort of financial support.

My sister Helen did establish a trust fund for the twins at Harris Bank in Hinsdale, and made the first donation herself. It was necessary for my wife and I to sign papers at the bank. We did so, however, only upon insistence from Helen and others. Most people never knew about the fund, and we made no attempt to promote it's existence. The maximum balance never reached $3000.

There were other monetary gifts which did not go into the trust fund. These were personal gifts to Sandi and I to use for the twins. All of these funds were used to purchase medical supplies, formula and baby clothes.

Receiving monetary gifts made us a little uneasy. Quite often, however, these gifts were accompanied by a note or letter, which I can best describe as warm and inspiring. We received a number of donations to the trust fund from retired individuals. The enclosed message, whether long or short, almost always contained the same theme. The individual was on a fixed income, could not afford to send much, but really wanted to help. He or she knew that our girls needed the money more than they did.

This support, while still considered monetary, was very special. I could understand, thanks to these wonderful people, what it means to "give til it hurts," and to "give of yourself."

These gifts also tended to include the offering of prayers for Megan and Shannon. To know that so many people cared so much about strangers, was heart-lifting. Each day, when I prayed for the recovery of our daughters, I also prayed for all of those who had given so freely.

There is no doubt, that the greatest support received by us, was the non-financial, non-physical variety. When it comes to this type, most people think of emotional support; having someone just being there, saying the right things. We certainly had a good amount of that. So many of our friends and relatives would ask us how things were going, and then would actually listen and reply. They were always concerned and positive, while, most of the time knowing just what to say.

This same type of support seemed to spread to strangers. Whenever anyone came to realize who we were and what our situation was, they had something good to say. We had said from the very beginning that this was a good story, a happy story. We now had a lot of other people believing the same thing, and helping us get through whatever difficult times we might see.

Sandi had received a phone call, late on the evening of March 25th. The caller identified herself as Georgia Welsh, the aunt of the Lakeberg twins. Since Sandi had been out of her room at the time, the nurse took a message to pass along.

Sandi was a little apprehensive about returning the call, but eventually decided it would be best for her to at least be polite. The following morning, she called Georgia back. As it turned out, she was glad she did. Georgia only wanted to wish us the best, and to let us know that their thoughts and prayers were with the twins. She said she would be there if we needed her.

Here was a representative of a family which had been, more or less, dragged through the media mud. Instead of looking for sympathy from us, however, Georgia was offering encouragement, prayers and even advise, should we desire it. Sandi greatly appreciated the conversation and Georgia's concern.

Prayer is a very personal thing to me. I normally don't speak about it, nor do I ask others to. My prayers are, most often, silent and to myself. Usually, I do not pray out loud, in front of others, except when participating in church services. Prayer has been virtually an everyday part of my life since early childhood. During our crisis situation with the twins, however, it became even more significant. I can honestly say that prayer, and the belief in God significantly helped us in our efforts to get through several very difficult situations in the past year. To anyone who doesn't believe in God, I can say I respect your belief (or lack of), but I think you should reconsider.

Sandi and I prayed together on many occasions, that our babies would be allowed to live and grow. There were others who had been praying for the same thing almost as long.

My mother, for instance, always had the ability to effect an outcome with prayer. At least, that's what it has seemed like to me. As soon as she knew of our situation, she began personal prayer and eventually took her intentions to the Catholic Church where she lives in Colorado. The situation was similar with Sandi's parents. They live in a retirement community in Englewood, Florida. The Presbyterian Church congregation was praying for our girls and their survival, long before most people knew they were conjoined.

That was just the beginning. Once we had appeared on national television, the amount of prayer support began to quickly multiply. We received phone calls and letters from our own area and out of state. So many people felt moved or compelled. One gentleman, here in Illinois, felt that he could best help by phoning me and explaining the amazing power of prayer. While I appreciated his efforts, it did seem like a bit much. His point, however, was well taken. In the right hands, there is no more powerful force than prayer; for it has, at it's command, the very power of God.

I received word from friends I had known in Canada, that a prayer chain had been started for the girls. In addition, someone in South Carolina assured us that their entire prayer community was focusing on the survival of Shannon and Megan.

Closer to home, our own Parish, as well as numerous

others in the diocese, were including the girls in their Sunday intentions. Many of the people we worked with reminded us daily, that their congregations were praying for the twins.

It was almost overwhelming. Each time I thought about it, a lump came to my throat. What would have happened without such support? What might happen now that such support was in place?

We realized that God doesn't always answer our prayers by providing exactly what is asked for. Often times, we find that his will has another purpose. We prayed to God therefore, that the purpose he had in allowing our daughters to go through what they had, coincided with what everyone else was asking for in their prayers. It was a long road to recovery. We hoped the prayers would continue at least until Megan and Shannon were happy and healthy young girls.

Effective support has many different aspects. One aspect would be represented by a couple of occurrences which took place just days after the separation surgery. When Sandi and I entered the girls room in NICU, we noticed there was a little knit object of some sort attached to each incubator. Further examination showed them to be two tiny pairs of booties, absolutely the smallest we had ever seen. Figuring one of the nurses was responsible, we asked where they had come from. The reply was, "we don't know." The nurse on duty held up an empty envelope addressed to Megan and Shannon Fanning at Children's Memorial Hospital. "They came in here," she said, "no letter, no return address, just the booties."

This may not seem like an awful lot, but to us it was

wonderful. Someone had cared enough to make these special little gifts. They didn't care about being recognized for, or complimented on, what they had done. They just quietly, anonymously did it. It gave us both a little boost that day.

Another event did also. There were, of course, many other children at the hospital when Megan and Shannon arrived. Some of them had been there for quite a while. Most of them had something fairly serious wrong with them. One little girl, must have heard through the grapevine about our girls. She made a hand drawn poster and had a nurse deliver it to the girls' room. It was just a poster like you would expect from a young, school age girl, but it was beautiful. Even though this child had her own problems, possibly as bad as or worse than the twins', she cared enough to make a little present and wish the girls well.

There was one additional incident I must include in the area of support. It involved two beautiful girls and a family who must have known, all too well, what we were going through.

A short time after the surgery, we received a letter from a family in Wisconsin. As we opened it, two photographs fell out. Sandi read the letter and I looked at the pictures. They were of two girls, who looked to be about 9 or 10 years old. They were slightly different, one appearing to be just a little heavier than the other. It was obvious, however, that they were twins. They were also, quite beautiful. Since I didn't recognize them, I assumed the family must have been friends of Sandi's. When she handed me the letter and I began reading, however, I realized it was a much different story.

I won't go into all of the details, but as it turned out, the girls in the photographs had been conjoined at birth. As a matter of fact, their situation had , apparently, been similar to our girls'.

The family had been kind enough to offer their support. They had been through it before and would be praying for us. Once again, we were thrilled. Another family, one that had known some of the same pain and had gone through some of the same emotional hardships, was offering whatever assistance they could. There were an awful lot of good people out there, and we were hearing from many of them.

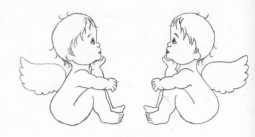

Chapter 16

Getting Better

The first few days and nights following the babies' homecoming, presented some special challenges. Even though Sandi and I were now able to spend more time at home, we found ourselves spending less time on certain activities. The greatest effect, regrettably, was on our ability to spend quality time with the other children. The twins required a lot of care, and we probably were also just a little paranoid about their welfare. Even with a standard nursery monitor setup so we could hear them cry, I found it quite difficult to fall asleep at night. I kept thinking that there would be no lights or buzzer to let us know if something should be seriously wrong.

It wasn't just at night either. During the daytime, I found myself periodically placing my face close to one or the other twin, to make sure their little hearts were beating and their lungs were working.

Sandi wasn't much better. She held them a lot whenever she could, and worried about them when they weren't in her arms. They were just so small, and had been through so much.

The mechanics of tube feeding were pretty simple, and presented no problem for Tanja or I. Sandi was still the expert, but we all helped out.

The baby "weigh-ins" were conducted at least once each day. After the first few days, we began to worry. Although we were feeding them the prescribed amount, neither baby was showing a weight gain. In addition, their bowel movements continued to be quite loose. This was despite regular doses of Paregoric.

Paregoric was one of the drugs both girls were receiving. It was used to slow down the movement of food through their digestive systems. Because their bowels were shorter than normal, and still healing, they were not processing food long enough to derive all of the nutrition required.

The loose movements concerned us greatly. With the use of Paregoric, we had expected more solid stools.

To add to these problems, both girls were poor sleepers, being awake numerous times each night, and not always satisfied with a diaper change and a feeding. It was evident to us that they were either uncomfortable or in pain. They also had, almost immediately, developed gastric problems.

We continued to monitor their weights closely, and discovered that the time and circumstances of the weigh-ins had a significant effect on the patterns. Apparently, when initially weighed at home, they had just eaten, and were relatively inactive. Because they were so small, the weight increase per day we were looking for was, actually, less than the weight of a single feeding. This meant that if they were currently being weighed with empty stomachs, it would take them several days to show an increase over that of the initial weigh-in.

We figured this out just as we were about to call Doctor Moss following the second no-gain day. Sure enough, the next morning both girls showed an increase.

We were able to rest a little easier, but not so Megan and Shannon. They continued to have gas problems. Their food formula's were changed several times before we found a combination they could tolerate.

It wasn't easy, but we were becoming used to their limited sleep, and tender tummies. Everyone was very much aware of the fact that we were living the best of the possible scenarios so far. We had no complaints.

The weeks went by rather slowly. We continued to hope and pray for the girls rapid progress. They seemed to be getting better alright, but it was a slow process.

Shannon was the first to lose her feeding tube. We had been bottle feeding them as much as possible, and she had caught on quicker than her sister. After four weeks, she was taking in enough calories for us to remove the tube.

Megan, on the other hand, was more of a problem. She did not want to be fed from the bottle, and most often drank very little. We tried every size, shape and texture of nipple, just in case that was the problem. While she did prefer a specific one, she still acted as though drinking through a nipple was just too much work for her. We were

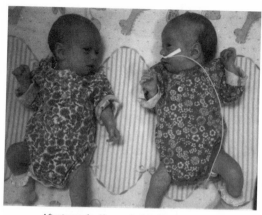

becoming quite worried about her. We realized that she was still receiving anti-seizure medication. That, in itself, would tend to make her a little lethargic. We knew that, if she continued to grow, and the dosages were not increased, she should become more fully alert and active. We hoped that her desire to drink on her own would also increase.

After ten weeks, Shannon had shed her feeding tube, while Megan still required hers.

In the meantime, we would continue to feed her through the tube only when absolutely necessary.

We had decided that, once the weather was nice and the twins were up to seeing a lot of people at one time, we would have them baptized. The services we had been to recently, had all been fairly long. This was at least partially due to the fact that any number of babies might be baptized a the same service. We were somewhat concerned, because the twins had not been anywhere outside of our home for more than a few minutes, and, if anything should go wrong with either of them, it would upset the service for all of the other families. When we called the parish to discuss a time and date, however, we were pleasantly surprised. Once they knew who we were, they offered to perform a private service. Sandi was quick to let them know we did not consider ourselves to be special, but they had their own reasons for wanting to baptize the twins separately.

They said the fact that we had been in the news and on television, would tend to detract from a multi-family service. They realized others would be curious about the girls, and might unintentionally make us feel uncomfortable. They also realized that we had not experienced a whole lot of privacy during the past few weeks, and they thought we could use some now. It was a gracious offer, and we eagerly accepted it.

So, on June 11th 1994, in a private Roman Catholic service, Megan and Shannon were baptized. All told, there were about twenty-five family members and close friends present.

Spring turned into Summer, and the girls continued their gradual improvement. The weather was nice and we were now able to take them out more often. Many people would stop and comment on our newborns, not realizing that they were actually several months old. A few others recognized us, and asked how the girls were doing.

All in all, life at home was beginning to be almost normal. By the time the twins were eleven weeks old, Megan had given up fighting us, and was reluctantly drinking from a bottle. Both girls had been back to the hospital several times for check-ups, with good results. The doctors were happy with their progress and increased the time between required visits. Megan had even been taken off of the anti-seizure medication.

Sandi and I, however, continued to worry about the them. Even though everything was going well, they were both still quite small, each weighing only about seven pounds at four months of age. In addition, their bowel movements continued to be quite loose.

The girls new pediatrician, Doctor Martine Nelson, was also rather pleased with their progress. She seemed to think they would catch up physically by the end of their first year. We thought they had a long way to go.

By the time summer was winding down, Doctor Nelson had given the go-ahead to begin working baby food into the girls diet. It was felt by all involved, that this would be the next big test for their intestinal tracts and digestive systems. Megan had finally mastered the art of bottle feeding. In fact, she was regularly drinking more than her sister, and accomplishing it faster.

The introduction of cereal was, at first, a disappointment. Like everything else new, it bothered both girls' tummies. Eventually, we did find a flavor and brand that both girls could tolerate. Megan took off quickly, not minding the feel of the different texture in her little mouth. Shannon, as we had now come to expect, was slower to accept it. She didn't really like anything non-liquid in her mouth.

At about the same time as this was taking place, both girls' cut their first tooth. In fact it happened to be the same tooth for each of them, coming through on the very same day. This was a happy sign. Except for their size, they were developing right on schedule.

The days continued to pass, and their feeding habits improved. Some fruits and vegetables were added to the previously all-cereal and formula diet. Shortly afterwards, when they had reached six and one half months, we had another happy surprise. Megan began to have solid bowel movements. It appeared as though that portion of her internals was working just fine.

Sandi and I had to laugh. Who would have thought we would get so excited about such bodily functions. We guessed that a lot of people, not knowing the circumstances, would have thought us to be rather weird. That didn't matter. Our reactions to such events may have made us appear weird, but such events themselves only made Megan or Shannon appear more normal.

A few days later, I happened to speak with Doctor Moss, who had moved and was living and working in New Mexico. He was happy to hear from us, and anxious for news of the girls.

His reactions were positive. When I brought him up to date on the girls, he was quite pleased. When I told him that they had begun to eat baby food, he asked about their bowel movements. There was noticeable concern in his voice after I told him that Shannon's were still loose. It was pretty easy to tell that he had hoped things would be more normal by then.

I finished the conversation by getting his new address and promising more pictures. After I hung up, I thought about his reaction. Should we be as concerned? I would certainly think so. It was obvious that Shannon's intestines were not working as well as her sisters. Maybe they never would.

Sandi and I made up our minds once and for all. It really didn't matter so much anymore. Our prayers had been answered to such a high degree already, that we couldn't be anything but happy and thankful.

God, through the miracle of modern medicine and exceptionally caring people, had given us our two beautiful daughters.

Those daughters were becoming active little girls. Of course there would be difficult times. What parents haven't seen their share? We were ready for whatever was to come. After all, wasn't it about time we starting treating the girls as we would want everyone else to treat them, as normal children?

The twins had, over the past few months, developed more and more of their own individual characteristics from a personality and behavioral standpoint. Curiously enough they had, during the same time period, rediscovered each other.

Shannon would, for minutes at a time, stare at her sister. In the meantime, Megan, having noticed Shannon's flying limbs, seemed to delight in grabbing on to whatever appendage she could reach.

Yes, they had certainly changed. No matter how we looked at it, however, they were still little angels. As Sandi and I sat together on the floor and watched our little girls play, we were reminded of the fact that, at one time, before that first ultrasound had shown two tiny heart beats, before this whole amazing episode had begun, they really were just one. God had chosen to split that one tiny egg and make it two. Two separate embryos to become our two separate angels.

I got up from the floor, and brought my thoughts back to the present.

"If you're okay here with the two of them, I think I'll go into the den and start working my way through all of the documentation we've gathered," I said.

Sandi had just begun changing Shannon's diaper. She smiled and nodded affirmation. "Do you think you might start writing again?" she asked.

"Yes," I said, "and I believe I've got just the right story. How does *Separated Angels* sound for a title?"

"I like it" she said. "Before you leave, though, you might want to have a look at this,"

She was, quite obviously, pointing at Shannon's diaper.

"What is it? What's the matter?" I asked.

She was grinning ear to ear when she responded, "Nothing, except that you could break a window with what she's done in there."

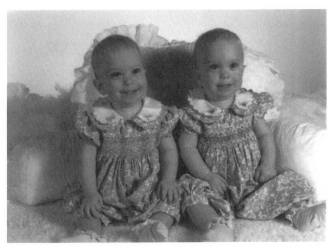

The twins as they appeared just prior to their first birthday.
Megan left, Shannon right.
Photo by CP Studios

Afterword

As time passes, the story of Megan and Shannon,
and their unusual birth, begins to fade.
They are now one year old; both are healthy and strong.
Except for the scars on their tummies, and the lack of belly
buttons, they cannot be distinguished from other
twins of a similar age.
They each have their own distinct personality.
Shannon is still the feisty one, and now outweighs her sister.
Megan is more gentle and loves to cuddle.
Sandi and I continue to thank all those who, in any way, helped
us during that tough year and a half. We also continue to thank
God for what he has given us.
For me, the past year has offered an ironic twist.
Within the four months prior to the celebration of the twins first
birthday, two of my own sisters celebrated their last.
The lord took two beautiful Fanning girls to be with him, and
gave us two beautiful Fanning girls in their places.
Sissy and Nettie we will miss you.